Ultrasound of the Diaphragm and the Respiratory Muscles

Ultrasound of the Diaphragm and the Respiratory Muscles

Edited by

Massimo Zambon
Anesthesiologist and Critical Care Specialist
Head of Department of Anesthesia and
Intensive Care of the Uboldo Hospital, Cernusco sul Naviglio, Milan, Italy

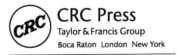

CRC Press
Taylor & Francis Group
Boca Raton London New York

CRC Press is an imprint of the
Taylor & Francis Group, an **informa** business

First edition published 2022
by CRC Press
6000 Broken Sound Parkway NW, Suite 300, Boca Raton, FL 33487-2742

and by CRC Press
2 Park Square, Milton Park, Abingdon, Oxon, OX14 4RN

© 2022 Taylor & Francis Group, LLC

CRC Press is an imprint of Taylor & Francis Group, LLC

Library of Congress Cataloging-in-Publication Data

Names: Zambon, Massimo, editor.
Title: Ultrasound of the diaphragm and the respiratory muscles / edited by
Massimo Zambon.
Description: Boca Raton, FL : CRC Press, 2022. | Includes bibliographical
references and index. | Summary: "Ultrasound is the most reliable,
easily available, fast, non-invasive technique to study diaphragm
function, and is an irreplaceable tool to diagnose, monitor and
follow-up critical respiratory patients. This essential guide analyzes
every aspect of ultrasound of the diaphragm which is vital to provide
the most suitable treatment"-- Provided by publisher.
Identifiers: LCCN 2021057518 (print) | LCCN 2021057519 (ebook) | ISBN
9780367652777 (hardback) | ISBN 9780367652760 (paperback) | ISBN
9781003128694 (ebook)
Subjects: MESH: Diaphragm--diagnostic imaging | Respiratory Tract
Diseases--diagnostic imaging | Respiration, Artificial
Classification: LCC QP145 (print) | LCC QP145 (ebook) | NLM WF 800 | DDC
611/.26--dc23/eng/20220106
LC record available at https://lccn.loc.gov/2021057518
LC ebook record available at https://lccn.loc.gov/2021057519

ISBN: 9780367652777 (hbk)
ISBN: 9780367652760 (pbk)
ISBN: 9781003128694 (ebk)

DOI: 10.1201/9781003128694

Typeset in Minion
by Deanta Global Publishing Services, Chennai, India

Access the Support Material: www.routledge.com/9780367652760

*To our teachers, colleagues, trainees, who have been a
source of knowledge and inspiration. And to all the patients,
hoping knowledge will help to improve their care.*

M.Z.

Contents

Preface

The diaphragm is the main respiratory muscle. Nevertheless, we can affirm that it has been the least monitored aspect of respiration in medical history, due to the lack of available tools and technologies to assess its function.

With the spreading use of ultrasound and the implementation of POCUS (Point of Care Ultrasound), some clinicians started to understand that a new "window" of opportunity was available to obtain information about the respiratory workload of our patients. Ultrasound of the diaphragm is the last piece of a puzzle that allows clinicians to assess the respiratory condition and to obtain valuable data of the patients with a quick, non-invasive, yet accurate tool.

To our knowledge, this is the first book entirely dedicated to the subject. The book is structured in four sections: a first part dedicated to the basics of anatomy, physiology, and ultrasound; a second part describing the technique, featuring illustrations and videoclips; and third and fourth parts dedicated to applications and new insights, respectively. Chapters are written by leading experts in the field from different countries, including Italy, the Netherlands, France, Brazil, Greece, and Canada. Given the relatively recent "discovery" of diaphragm ultrasound, this choice has allowed us to approach the subject from different points of view to provide a comprehensive perspective. My deep gratitude goes to every author of each chapter; without their contribution the goal would have been impossible to achieve.

Massimo Zambon

Editor

Dr Massimo Zambon is a skilled anesthesiologist and critical care specialist, Head of the Department of Anesthesia and Intensive Care of the Uboldo Hospital in Cernusco sul Naviglio, Milan. Graduated in medicine at the University of Trieste before settling in Italy, he gained professional experience working in some of the major European hospitals both as researcher (research fellow at Erasme Hospital in Brussels, Belgium, 2005–06) and clinician (anesthesiologist and critical care specialist at La Pitié-Salpétrière Hospital in Paris, France, 2007–08). Subsequently, he became full-time staff physician at San Raffaele Hospital in Milan, Italy (2009–15), where he was involved in training activities for internal staff, residents, and students of the San Raffaele University. He has wide-ranging expertise in intensive care medicine, mainly focusing on the application of ultrasound in critically ill patients. In the last decade, he has started to perform ultrasound of the diaphragm on critically ill patients, an innovative and non-invasive tool that facilitates assess to respiratory muscle function. He has published more than 20 papers in critical care indexed journals, mostly focused on ultrasound, and a number of abstracts and book chapters.

List of Contributors

Andre L. P. de Albuquerque
Pulmonary Division, University of São Paulo
Research Institute, Hospital Sirio Libanes
São Paulo, Brazil

Elena Bignami
Department of Medicine and Surgery
University of Parma
Parma, Italy

Gianmaria Cammarota
Department of Medicine and Surgery
University of Perugia
Perugia, Italy

Leticia Z. Cardenas
Intensive Care Unit,
AC Camargo Cancer Center
São Paulo, Brazil

Cristian Deana
Department of Anesthesia and Intensive Care
University Hospital of Udine
Udine, Italy

Heder J. de Vries
Department of Intensive Care Medicine
Amsterdam UMC, Location VUmc
Amsterdam, the Netherlands

Martin Dres
Service de Médecine Intensive et Réanimation
Hôpital Pitie Salpetriere, APHP
Sorbonne University
Paris, France.

Abdallah Fayssoil
Hopital Raymond Poincaré
Université de Versailles SQY
Garches, France

Quentin Fossé
Service de Médecine Intensive et Réanimation
Hôpital Pitié Salpétrière, APHP
Paris, France

Marco Gemma
NeuroAnesthesia and Intensive Care
Fondazione IRCCS Istituto Neurologico C. Besta
Milan, Italy

Mark E. Haaksma
Department of Intensive Care Medicine
Amsterdam UMC, Location VUmc
Amsterdam, the Netherlands

Leo Heunks
Department of Intensive Care Medicine
Amsterdam UMC, Location VUmc
Amsterdam, the Netherlands

Annemijn H. Jonkman
Department of Intensive Care Medicine
Amsterdam UMC, Location VUmc
Amsterdam, the Netherlands

Daniele Orso
Department of Medicine
University of Udine
Udine, Italy

Pauliane V. Santana
Intensive Care Unit
AC Camargo Cancer Center
São Paulo, Brazil

Savvoula Savvidou
ICU Department
Papageorgiou General Hospital
Thessaloniki, Greece

Annia Schreiber
Interdepartmental Division of Critical
Care Medicine
University of Toronto
Toronto, Canada
and
Keenan Research Center and Li Ka Shing
Knowledge Institute
Unity Health Toronto (St Michael's
Hospital)
Toronto, Canada

Zhonghua Shi
Department of Intensive Care Medicine
Amsterdam UMC, Location VUmc
Amsterdam, the Netherlands

Eleni Soilemezi
ICU Department
Papageorgiou General Hospital
Thessaloniki, Greece

Panagiota Sotiriou
ICU Department
Papageorgiou General Hospital
Thessaloniki, Greece

Matthew Tsagourias
ICU Department
Papageorgiou General Hospital
Thessaloniki, Greece

Pieter R. Tuinman
Department of Intensive Care Medicine
Amsterdam UMC, Location VUmc
Amsterdam, the Netherlands

Luigi Vetrugno
Department of Medicine
University of Udine
Udine, Italy

Myrte Wennen
Department of Intensive Care Medicine
Amsterdam UMC, Location VUmc
Amsterdam, the Netherlands

Massimo Zambon
Department of Anesthesia and Intensive
Care
Ospedale di Cernusco sul Naviglio – ASST
Melegnano e Martesana,
Milan, Italy

Part I

Introduction

Anatomy, Physiology, and Dysfunction of the Diaphragm

Marco Gemma

In evolution, the diaphragm muscle is unique to mammals, and its physiological importance cannot be argued (1).

Anatomy

The diaphragm is a dome-shaped 2–4 mm thick muscular sheet that separates the thoracic and the abdominal cavities (2–5) (Figure 1.1).

Actually, the diaphragm is formed by two muscle bellies (*domes* or *cupolae*) connected at the level of the xiphosternal joint by the *central tendon*. This flat non-contractile collagen aponeurosis provides support to the heart, whereas the right and the left cupolae support the corresponding lungs. The apex of the diaphragm ranges widely in height during the breathing cycle (even between the fourth rib and the costal margin) depending on breathing depth, body posture, and abdominal pressure. The right cupola, lying above the liver, reaches a 2–3 cm higher level than the left one.

The diaphragm muscle fibres arise from the inner aspect of the thoracic cage (4–9).

Posteriorly, the diaphragm muscle fibres are organized in two paired *crura*, which originate from the anterior aspects of L1–L3 and are joined by the *median arcuate ligament*. Hypertrophy or lower displacement of this fibrous structure may cause the *median arcuate ligament syndrome* (MALS, also known as *celiac artery compression syndrome, celiac axis syndrome, celiac trunk compression syndrome,* or *Dunbar syndrome*).

More anteriorly, the diaphragm muscle fibres rise from the paired *medial arcuate ligaments*, which join the vertebral tendinous origin of the respective diaphragmatic crus to the transverse processes of L1 or L2, after covering the anterior surface of the major psoas muscle. Even more anteriorly, the muscle fibres take origin from the paired *lateral arcuate ligaments*, which spread from the transverse processes of T12–L3 (variably) to the mid portion of the twelfth ribs covering the quadratus lumborum muscle. All these

DOI: 10.1201/9781003128694-2

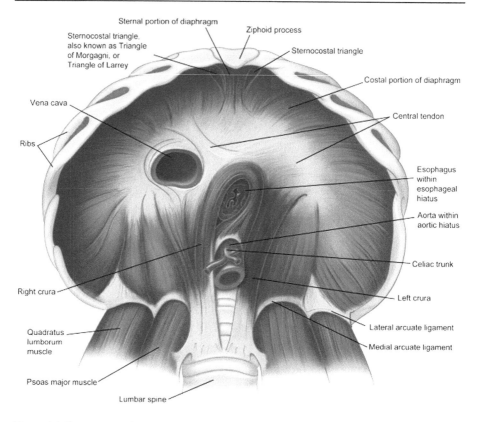

Figure 1.1 The anatomy of the normal diaphragm. Reproduced with permission from ref. 4 (Downey R, Anatomy of the normal diaphragm, *Thorac Surg Clin* 21(2) (2011) 273–79). Anatomy of the diaphragm

arcuate ligaments are thickened fascial bands that are sometimes mistaken for pathological structures on clinical imaging.

Antero-laterally and anteriorly, the cupolae are formed by muscle fibres originating from the inner surface of the lower six ribs and of the xiphoid process, respectively.

From their origin inside the rib cage the diaphragm muscle fibres direct cephalad and are substantially vertical. They gradually horizontalize, producing the aforementioned dome shape of the muscle. In this setting, the distal part of the diaphragmatic dome abuts the lower rib cage from the costal insertion to a point referred to as *costophrenic angle*. This portion is known as the zone of apposition (ZOA) (10, 11).

During quiet breathing the ZOA is one-quarter to one-third of the total inner rib cage area.

A number of ligaments connect the diaphragm to neighbouring viscera (5).

The *inferior pulmonary ligament*, the *phrenopericardial ligament*, the *falciform* and the paired *triangular ligaments* of the liver, the *phrenicoesophageal ligament*, and the *phrenicocolic ligament* (to the angle of the ascending colon) are pleural, pericardial, or peritoneal thickening.

The ligament of Treitz is made up of muscle fibres from the left crus reaching the duodenojejunal angle.

Three hiatuses allow passage between the thoracic and the abdominal cavities (5, 12).

The *caval hiatus*, at the T8 level, in the middle of the central tendon, is traversed by the inferior vena cava and some branches of the right phrenic nerve. It enlarges during inspiration, favouring blood flow to the heart.

The *oesophageal hiatus*, at the T10 level, through the right crus, allows passage to the oesophagus, the vagus nerve, and some sympathetic nerve branches. It works as a muscular sphincter, constricting during inspiration and preventing gastroesophageal reflux.

The *aortic hiatus*, at the T12 level, beyond the crura, transmits the aorta, the thoracic duct and the azygos and hemiazygos veins. It is unaffected by diaphragmatic contraction.

Several smaller and inconstant apertures in the diaphragm allow the passage of blood and lymph vessels.

The superior surface of the diaphragm receives its blood supply from branches of the *internal thoracic mammary artery* (the *musculophrenic, pericardiacophrenic*, and *superior epigastric arteries*) and of the *lower thoracic aorta* (*phrenic branches*), besides. the lower five *intercostal and subcostal arteries*.

The inferior surface is supplied by branches of the *abdominal aorta* or of the *coeliac trunk* (*inferior phrenic arteries*) (5).

The venous drainage strictly mirrors the arterial supply. Eventually the superior surface veins drain into the *internal thoracic vein* and the inferior surface veins drain into the *inferior vena cava* (right hemidiaphragm) and the *renal* or *suprarenal left vein* (left hemidiaphragm).

Both diaphragmatic surfaces are covered by lymph plexuses anastomosing with each other and with pleural and peritoneal lymphatics. Retrosternal, perioesophageal/caval, and periaortic lymph nodes receive the lymphatic drainage, respectively, from the anterior, middle, and posterior third of the diaphragm (5).

Motor innervation comes to the diaphragm exclusively through the paired *phrenic nerves*. Except for a small contribution from the *sixth or seventh intercostal nerves*, the phrenic nerves provide also the sensitive innervation (5, 13–15).

The phrenic nerves rise from the ventral horn (lamina IX) of C3–C5. They reach the diaphragm laterally to the inferior vena cava on the right and laterally to the heart on the left and then divide in several branches inside the muscle thickness. The innervation of the two hemidiaphragms is ipsilateral and even the crural fibres are supplied by the ipsilateral phrenic nerve, regardless of their side of origin but according to their course to the right or left of the oesophageal opening. The innervation is somatotopic, since more rostral medullary segments innervate more ventral diaphragmatic portions (16, 17).

The phrenic motor neurons are monosynaptically innervated by pre-motor neurons lying in the *ventro-lateral* and *dorso-medial medulla* and descending ipsilaterally along the *ventro-lateral* and *ventro-medial funiculi*. These pre-motor neurons receive excitatory and inhibitory inputs from different nuclei in the medulla itself, generating the "pacing" of breathing (the *pre-Boetzinger complex* drives inspiration, the *Boetzinger complex* the scalhift to expiration, the *retrotrapezoid nucleus* active expiration). The complex and still incompletely understood control of such respiratory drive nuclei by the cerebral cortex and by central and peripheral chemo- and mechano-receptors goes beyond the scope of this text (1, 18).

The development of the diaphragm occurs during weeks 4–12 of embryogenesis and is the result of the fusion of four primitive structures (transverse septum, pleuroperitoneal folds, oesophageal mesentery, and muscular body wall). Defects in fusion give rise to congenital diaphragmatic hernias such as the *anterior (Morgagni) hernia*, accounting for around 10%

of cases, and the *posterior (Bochdalek) hernia*, accounting for around 90% of cases and more common on the left side (19).

Physiology

The diaphragm is the main muscle responsible for spontaneous ventilation (Video 1.1).

During inspiration its muscle fibres shorten. This contraction makes the cupolae descend and the ZOA decrease. During quiet breathing in a normal upright adult, the dome descends with inspiration about 2 cm and does not change in shape. The ZOA reduces accordingly and may be absent at total lung capacity.

The trans-diaphragmatic pressure developed during inspiration is mechanically determined by the Laplace's law, being directly proportional to the tension produced by the contracting muscle fibres and inversely proportional to the thoracic cross-sectional area.

The resulting increment in abdominal pressure displaces the ventral abdominal wall outward. Nevertheless, this increment in abdominal pressure, together with the presence of rather fixed and incompressible abdominal viscera, provides a fulcrum on which diaphragm contraction acts to raise the lower ribs in the well-known *bucket-handle* rib movement. This is the so-called *insertional component* of the inspiratory action of the diaphragm. A second component (*appositional component*) is the abdominal pressure itself as it is produced over the ZOA, which is transmitted to the lower rib cage and expands it.

A third component of the inspiratory action of the diaphragm is the negative pressure produced in the thoracic cavity by the lower displacement of the cupolae. This component would produce an inward movement of the upper rib cage that is prevented by the action of the intercostal and scalene muscles (5, 20, 21).

This inspiratory mechanics in the upper rib cage does not change significantly between the upright and the supine position. Conversely, the lower rib cage expands much less in the supine than in the upright posture and may even move inwards in cases of absent abdominal and intercostal muscle tone, e.g., in tetraplegic patients (22). This is related to the cephalad displacement of the abdominal content, which reduces the anterior ZOA and lengthen the diaphragmatic muscle, so that the axial tension, normally produced in the upright posture, is converted to a radial tension.

Another critical issue determining the effectiveness of the diaphragm contraction is lung volume. As the lung volume increases, the ZOA decreases and both the insertional and the appositional components of the diaphragm inspiratory action lose effectiveness. Moreover, as the lung volume increases, the trans-diaphragmatic pressure generated by the diaphragm contraction decreases almost linearly. This is due to the lengthening of the muscle fibres, which places them on a less advantageous portion of the length vs tension curve, and to the increasing radius of curvature of the cupolae (cf Laplace's law) (22). Such an effect of lung volume is physiologically present throughout the normal breathing cycle as the lungs inflate and deflate, but is also at stake in common diseases such as COPD with its well-known increase in lung volume.

Video 1.1 Diaphragm movement during respiration

The diaphragm relaxes during expiration as, thanks to their elastic properties, the cupolae return to their initial length and tension (5, 23–25). Relaxation abnormalities play a role in reducing diaphragmatic performance. For example, the sarcoplasmic reticulum Ca^{++} pump efficiency is reduced with increasing age.

From a mechanical point of view, diaphragm relaxation occurs in two consecutive phases, an isotonic relaxation (lengthening), followed by an isometric relaxation (tension decay). Although important in *in vitro* studies, this concept is poorly relevant *in vivo*, a setting in which the curve of the trans-diaphragmatic pressure decay is the common tool to evaluate diaphragm activity. Two variables describe such a curve yielding clinically significant information. The first one is the *Maximum Relaxation Rate (MRR)*, which is the lowest (most negative) derivative of the pressure vs time function. The second is the *Time Constant* of the latter part of the curve, which is normally mono-exponential. Slowing of inspiratory diaphragm relaxation is an index of diaphragm fatigue and is recorded as an MMR decrease and a Time Constant increase.

Diaphragm relaxation is critical for the subsequent inspiratory function itself. In fact diaphragm contraction depends also on the resting length of the muscle fibres. The optimal resting length is around the functional residual capacity (FRC) (26). Incomplete relaxation, i.e., incomplete expiration, poses the lungs and the diaphragm in the less advantageous portions of the lung compliance curve and of the length/tension curve, respectively.

Moreover, diaphragmatic blood supply is warranted during relaxation but it is significantly reduced during contraction (actually it can be abolished during extremely forceful contraction) due to the ensuing intramuscular pressure. This pattern – resembling coronary circulation – contributes to diaphragmatic fatigue in cases of delayed or slowed relaxation, particularly at high breathing rates, in a deleterious feedback (5, 27–29).

Forceful contraction of the diaphragm is not unique to pathological states producing airway obstruction. In fact the respiratory function of the diaphragm is not limited to inspiration/expiration. In fact the diaphragm contributes to the so-called *expulsive behaviour* in a coordinated activity with laryngeal structures: this encompasses coughing, expectoration, and sternutation, complex activities meant at *clearing and protecting* the airways.

Actually, the diaphragm muscle is composed by four types of motor units, like other skeletal muscles: the slow (S), the fast resistant (FR), the fast intermediate (FI), and the fast fatigable (FF) motor units, which differ in progressively higher diameter, higher velocity of shortening, greater force production, and lower fatigue resistance. This is due to different isomeric expression of myosin heavy chains and different rate of ATP hydrolysis of their constituent fibres. Motor units are recruited in an orderly fashion: S and FR motor units are recruited first, to accomplish lower force, high duty breathing activity. Expulsive behaviour requires powerful, short-duration contraction, which allows sufficient time for fatigue recovery by FI and FF units (1, 30).

There is evidence that sarcopenia related to ageing or chronic disease selectively affects FI and FF. This explains why these conditions are in their first stage accompanied by expulsive behaviour alterations rather than respiratory failure (31–33).

Recently, attention developed about non-respiratory functions of the diaphragm (2).

The crura may have a poor role in inspiration, acting rather on the esophagus as an anti-reflux barrier and entering the complex mechanisms of swallowing and vomiting. The latter requires also modulation of the intra-abdominal pressure, which is heavily influenced by diaphragmatic contraction as a whole and is involved in many different tasks such as micturition, defecation, parturition, and in even more complex tasks such as phonation. Moreover, a possible role of the diaphragmatic control on intra-abdominal pressure in stabilizing the spine has been particularly evaluated by the osteopathic literature (*postural function* of the diaphragm).

Dysfunction

From a functional point of view, the diaphragm activity may be impaired by weakness, paralysis, or eventration. Commonly, the latter involves only a portion of one hemidiaphragm, while weakness and paralysis involve an entire hemidiaphragm or the whole diaphragm.

Unilateral (hemidiaphragmatic) involvement is usually asymptomatic and is evidenced incidentally or as a precipitating factor of dyspnea during exercise or concomitant disease, particularly in the supine position (34, 35).

Bilateral involvement is most often symptomatic and accompanied by anamnestic clues (34, 36). Symptoms – exacerbated by exercise, supine position, and water immersion above the waist – consist in tachypnea and dyspnea accompanied by evident accessory respiratory muscles activity. Abdominal paradox (the abdomen moves inward as the rib cage expands during inspiration) is a hallmark of a weak or paralyzed diaphragm moving cephalad as the accessory inspiratory muscles lower the pleural pressure (34, 36). Sleep disorders are also frequent in this setting (37). Actually, impairment of the expulsive behaviour may be a predominant problem in chronic or subacute diaphragmatic dysfunctions, leading to pulmonary atelectasis and impaired clearance of secretions that ultimately favour respiratory failure.

Diaphragmatic dysfunction occurs as the result of many different conditions and both its natural history and its treatment options vary widely according to its etiology (Figure 1.2).

Traumatic, hemorrhagic, or neoplastic injuries to the medulla or the cervical spinal cord have an acute or subacute onset and may cause permanent diaphragmatic paralysis. Mechanical ventilation is required in around 40% of C3 lesions and in less than 15% of C4–C5 lesions (37).

Diseases affecting the lower motor neurons (e.g., amyotrophic lateral sclerosis, poliomyelitis, syringomyelia, paraneoplastic motor neuropathies, and spinal muscular atrophies) have a more variable history and are often characterized by diaphragmatic weakness progressively contributing to respiratory failure, whereas this rarely occurs in multiple sclerosis (34, 38).

The phrenic nerves may be mechanically damaged by direct trauma or by pulmonary or mediastinal neoplasms, but more often they are affected by iatrogenic trauma during cardiothoracic or neck surgery. Local hypothermia induced during cardiac surgery is a common cause of phrenic nerve stupor (39–41).

Inflammatory disorders due to autoimmunity (e.g., Guillain–Barré syndrome, which requires mechanical ventilation in 25% of cases, or neuralgic amyotrophy (Parsonage–Turner syndrome)) or infections (e.g., herpes zoster or Lyme disease) are other causes of diaphragm weakness or paralysis (42).

Partial or complete healing of phrenic nerve damage occurs often but commonly requires a long time (up to 3 years) (43, 44). Idiopathic or more clearly defined (e.g., chronic inflammatory demyelinating polyneuropathy and Charcot–Marie–Tooth disease) peripheral neuropathies follow their clinical course.

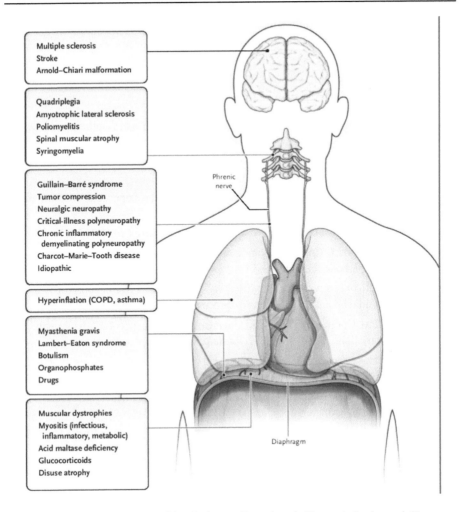

Multiple sclerosis
Stroke
Arnold–Chiari malformation

Quadriplegia
Amyotrophic lateral sclerosis
Poliomyelitis
Spinal muscular atrophy
Syringomyelia

Guillain–Barré syndrome
Tumor compression
Neuralgic neuropathy
Critical-illness polyneuropathy
Chronic inflammatory
 demyelinating polyneuropathy
Charcot–Marie–Tooth disease
Idiopathic

Hyperinflation (COPD, asthma)

Myasthenia gravis
Lambert–Eaton syndrome
Botulism
Organophosphates
Drugs

Muscular dystrophies
Myositis (infectious,
 inflammatory, metabolic)
Acid maltase deficiency
Glucocorticoids
Disuse atrophy

Phrenic
nerve

Diaphragm

Figure 1.2 Causes of dysfunction of the diaphragm. Reproduced with permission from ref. 35 (McCool FD, Tzelepis GE. Dysfunction of the diaphragm, *N Engl J Med*. 366 (2012) 932–42)

More distally in the neuromuscular path, alterations of the neuromuscular junction or of the muscle itself typically cause diaphragmatic weakness. This may occur occasionally and repeatedly (as in myasthenia gravis crisis, botulism, or organophosphate intoxication) or progressively in early or in adult life, as in some inherited or acquired myopathies (45, 46).

Ageing – as mentioned above – produces sarcopenia in a more systemic context and this usually affects the diaphragm (31–33).

The intensive care theatre is another setting in which diaphragmatic weakness occurs because of systemic conditions. In this setting, diaphragmatic hypotrophy ensues and is favoured by sepsis, multiorgan failure, hyperglycemia, muscle relaxants, and mechanical ventilation itself (even for brief periods). This is usually considered a consequence of critical-illness polyneuropathy and myopathy and has a multifactorial origin. In fact, besides simple diaphragmatic disuse, several conditions contribute to muscle atrophy hypophosphatemia, hypomagnesemia, hypokalemia, hypocalcemia, and thyroid disturbances. This issue is clinically prominent, since diaphragmatic hypotrophy prolongs ventilator dependency and its extent conditions the probability of weaning (47–49).

References

1. Fogarty MJ, Mantilla CB, Sieck GC. Breathing: motor control of diaphragm muscle. *Physiology* 2018;33:113–26.

2. Kocjan J, Adamek M, Gzik-Zroska B, et al. Network of breathing. Multifunctional role of the diaphragm: a review. *Adv Respir Med* 2017;85:224–32.

3. Nason LK, Walker CM, McNeeley MF, et al. Imaging of the diaphragm: anatomy and function. *Radiographics* 2012;32:E51–70.

4. Downey R. Anatomy of the normal diaphragm. *Thorac Surg Clin* 2011;21:273–9.

5. Shin MS, Berland LL. Computed tomography of retrocrural spaces: normal, anatomic variants, and pathologic conditions. *Am J Roentgenol* 1985;145:81–6.

6. Deviri E, Nathan H, Luchansky E. Medial and lateral arcuate ligaments of the diaphragm: attachment to the transverse process. *Anat Anz* 1988;166:63–7.

7. Silverman PM, Cooper C, Zeman RK. Lateral arcuate ligaments of the diaphragm: anatomic variations at abdominal CT. *Radiology.* 1992;185:105–8.

8. Lindner HH, Kemprud E. A clinicoanatomical study of the arcuate ligament of the diaphragm. *Arch Surg* 1971;103:600–5.

9. Horton KM, Talamini MA, Fishman EK. Median arcuate ligament syndrome: evaluation with CT angiography. *RadioGraphics* 2005;25:1177–82.

10. Loring SH, Mead J. Action of the diaphragm on the rib cage inferred from a force-balance analysis. *J Appl Physiol* 1982;53:756–60.

11. Goldman MD, Mead J. Mechanical interaction between the diaphragm and rib cage. *J Appl Physiol* 1973;35:197–204.

12. Panicek DM, Benson CB, Gottlieb RH, et al. The diaphragm: anatomic, pathologic, and radiologic considerations. *RadioGraphics* 1988;8:385–425.

13. Fell SC. Surgical anatomy of the diaphragm and the phrenic nerve. *Chest Surg Clin N Am* 1998;8:281–94.

14. Merendino KA, Johnson RJ, Skinner HH, et al. The intradiaphragmatic distribution of the phrenic nerve with particular reference to the placement of diaphragmatic incisions and controlled segmental paralysis. *Surgery* 1956;39:189–98.

15. Muller N, Volgyesi L, Bryan MH, et al. Diaphragmatic muscle tone. *J Appl Physiol* 1979;47:279–84.

16. Keswani NH, Hollinshead WH. The phrenic nucleus. III. Organization of the phrenic nucleus in the spinal cord of the cat and man. *Proc Staff Meet Mayo Clin* 1955;30:566–77.

17. Sieck GC, Roy RR, Powell P, et al. Muscle fiber type distribution and architecture of the cat diaphragm. *J Appl Physiol Respir Environ Exerc Physiol* 1983;55:1386–92.

18. Richter DW. Generation and maintenance of the respiratory rhythm. *J Exp Biol* 1982;100:93–107.

19. Taylor GA, Atalabi OM, Estroff JA. Imaging of congenital diaphragmatic hernias. *Pediatr Radiol* 2009;39:1–16.

20. Mortola JP, Sant'Ambrogio G. Motion of the rib cage and the abdomen in tetraplegic patients. *Clin Sci Mol Med* 1978;54:25–32.

21. Tusiewicz K, Moldofsky H, Bryan AC, et al. Mechanics of the rib cage and diaphragm during sleep. *J Appl Physiol* 1977;43:600–2.

22. Danon J, Druz WS, Goldberg NB, Sharp JT. Function of the isolated paced diaphragm and the cervical accessory muscles in C1 quadriplegics. *Am Rev Respir Dis* 1979;119: 909–19.

23. Coirault C, Chemla D, Lecarpentier Y. Relaxation of diaphragm muscle. *J Appl Physiol* 1999;87:1243–52.

24. Coirault C, Chemla D, Pery N, et al. Mechanical determinants of isotonic relaxation in isolated diaphragm muscle. *J Appl Physiol* 1993;75:2265–72.

25. Coirault C, Chemla D, Pery-Man N, et al. Isometric relaxation of isolated diaphragm muscle: influences of load, length, time and stimulation. *J Appl Physiol* 1994;766:1468–75.

26. Margulies SS, Farkas GA, Rodarte JR. Effects of body position and lung volume on in situ operating length of the canine diaphragm. *J Appl Physiol* 1990;69:1702–8.

27. Bellemare F, Wight D, Lavigne CM, et al. Effect of tension and timing of contraction on the blood flow of the diaphragm. *J Appl Physiol* 1983;54:1597–606.

28. Wait JL, Johnson RL. Patterns of shortening and thickening of the human diaphragm. *J Appl Physiol* 1997;83:1123–32.

29. Hu F, Comtois A, Grassino AE. Optimal diaphragmatic blood perfusion. *J Appl Physiol* 1992; 72:149–57.

30. Mantilla CB, Sieck GC. Phrenic motor unit recruitment during ventilatory and non-ventilatory behaviors. *Respir Physiol Neurobiol* 2011;179:57–63.

31. Elliott JE, Greising SM, Mantilla CB, et al. Functional impact of sarcopenia in respiratory muscles. *Respir Physiol Neurobiol* 2016;226:137–46.

32. Polkey MI, Harris ML, Hughes PD, et al. The contractile properties of the elderly human diaphragm. *Am J Respir Crit Care Med* 1997;155:1560–4.

33. Tolep K, Higgins N, Muza S, et al. Comparison of diaphragm strength between healthy adult elderly and young men. *Am J Respir Crit Care Med* 1995;152:677–82.

34. McCool FD, Tzelepis GE. Dysfunction of the diaphragm. *N Engl J Med* 2012;366:932–42.

35. Art N, Nickol AH, Cramer D, et al. Effect of severe isolated unilateral and bilateral diaphragm weakness on exercise performance. *Am J Respir Crit Care Med* 2002;165:1265–70.

36. Laghi F, Tobin MJ. Disorders of the respiratory muscles. *Am J Respir Crit Care Med* 2003;168:10–48.

37. Wicks AB, Menter RR. Long-term outlook in quadriplegic patients with initial ventilator dependency. *Chest* 1986;90:406–10.

38. Howard RS, Wiles CM, Hirsch NP, et al. Respiratory involvement in multiple sclerosis. *Brain* 1992;115:479–94.

39. Piehler JM, Pairolero PC, Gracey DR, et al. Unexplained diaphragmatic paralysis: a harbinger of malignant disease? *J Thorac Cardiovasc Surg* 1982;84:861–4.

40. Diehl JL, Lofaso F, Deleuze P, et al. Clinically relevant diaphragmatic dysfunction after cardiac operations. *J Thorac Cardiovasc Surg* 1994;107:487–98.

41. Merino-Ramirez MA, Juan G, Ramón M, et al. Electrophysiologic evaluation of phrenic nerve and diaphragm function after coronary bypass surgery: prospective study of diabetes and other risk factors. *J Thorac Cardiovasc Surg* 2006;132:530–6.

42. van Doorn PA, Ruts L, Jacobs BC. Clinical features, pathogenesis, and treatment of Guillain-Barré syndrome. *Lancet Neurol* 2008;7:939–50.

43. Summerhill EM, El-Sameed YA, Glidden TJ, et al. Monitoring recovery from diaphragm paralysis with ultrasound. *Chest* 2008;133:737–43.

44. Hughes PD, Polkey MI, Moxham J, et al. Long-term recovery of diaphragm strength in neuralgic amyotrophy. *Eur Respir J* 1999;13:379–84.

45. Mier-Jedrzejowicz A, Brophy C, Moxham J, et al. Assessment of diaphragm weakness. *Am Rev Respir Dis* 1988;137:877–83.

46. Gibson GJ. Diaphragmatic paresis: pathophysiology, clinical features, and investigation. *Thorax* 1989;44:960–70.

47. Chawla J, Gruener G. Management of critical illness polyneuropathy and myopathy. *Neurol Clin* 2010;28:961–77.

48. McParland C, Resch EF, Krishnan B, et al. Inspiratory muscle weakness in chronic heart failure: role of nutrition and electrolyte status and systemic myopathy. *Am J Respir Crit Care Med* 1995;151:1101–7.

49. Zambon M, Beccaria P, Matsuno J, et al. Mechanical ventilation and diaphragmatic atrophy in critically ill patients: an ultrasound study. *Crit Care Med* 2016;44:1347–52.

2

Ultrasound Basics

Massimo Zambon

One of the greatest advances in modern medicine is the possibility to obtain accurate imaging of internal organs and tissues, something that was once limited to examinations at autopsy.

Of all imaging techniques, ultrasound is by far the most increasingly used, because it is easily available, non-invasive, cost-effective, fast, and it allows either static or dynamic studies. Small, portable ultrasound machines are becoming "the stethoscopes of the future", allowing to explore almost every human body district from large organs (heart, liver, kidneys, lungs) until the smallest structures (such as intravascular ultrasound).

In the last decade, more and more research interest has focused on the function of the respiratory muscles, mainly the diaphragm.

A complete overview of ultrasound physics is beyond the purpose of this book. Nevertheless, to understand and to be able to perform any ultrasound assessment is essential to know how to set the machine and to understand how the machine works. A basic knowledge of the principles and basic concepts of ultrasound imaging is fundamental *to understand its clinical* applications. Furthermore, understanding the limitations of the technique allows to reduce image distortion and artefacts, thus reducing the chance of misdiagnosis.

The final purpose is to be able to obtain the best image possible and to interpret correctly the information acquired.

Sound is vibration of a physical medium. In clinical ultrasound, a mechanical vibrator, known as **the transducer**, is placed in contact with a surface (i.e., the skin, but it can be an internal surface such as the oesophagus) to create tissue vibrations (**sound waves**). The core of every transducer consists of piezoelectric crystals. Piezoelectricity is the process of using crystals to convert mechanical energy into electrical energy, or vice versa. Therefore, a transducer converts (or transduces) electrical energy to or from mechanical energy. The amplitudes of the returning echoes are represented as pixels of varying brightness along the vertical axis of the display. The brightness correlates with the strength of the returning signal.

Sound waves are often described as sinusoidal waves which are characterized by three properties (Figure 2.1):

- The *velocity* (V): the travel velocity or propagation velocity is determined solely by the medium through which it passes. For example, the speed of sound in soft tissues is approximately 1500m/s (Table 2.1).
- The *wavelength* (λ): the distance between two identical points on adjacent cycles.
- The *frequency* (f): number of wave repetitions per second (in Hertz, Hz).

The three properties are related by the formula: (Figure 2.1)

$$V = \lambda \cdot f$$

Interactions of Sound and Tissues

As ultrasound is generated by the transducer, its propagation through the body depends on its interactions with the tissues encountered. The interpretation of ultrasound images involves the recognition of many circumstances wherein information may be hidden or distorted by the physical interaction of ultrasound waves with tissue.

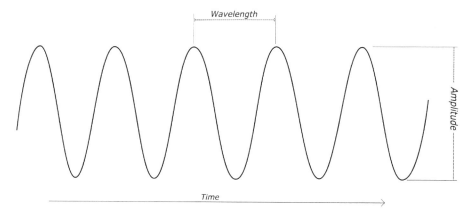

Figure 2.1 Propagation of sound waves

Table 2.1 Velocity of ultrasound in human tissues

Tissues	Velocity (m/s)
Bone	2–4000
Blood	1570
Water	1520
Fat	1450
Air	300

The interactions can be summarized in

1. *Reflection.* When a sound wave that propagates through a tissue reaches another tissue with different acoustic properties, at the interface between the two, a part of the ultrasound energy can be reflected back to the transducer, while the remaining part is transmitted through deeper structures.

    To understand how the ultrasound beam will be reflected vs. transmitted, the concept of *acoustic impedance* (Z) should be taken into account. Acoustic impedance is mainly related to the *density* (ρ) of the material and the velocity of ultrasound in the tissue (*v*).

$$Z = \rho \cdot v$$

    Notably, denser materials such as bone and fluids easily transmit ultrasound, whereas lung tissue and air are poor transmitters (Table 2.1).

    The reflection of sound is also greatly affected by the surface of the tissue. Smooth surfaces such as pleural, peritoneum, or pericardial membranes create *specular* reflection, acting like an acoustic mirror. The reflection is maximal when the angle of incidence is 90° (Figure 2.2a), whereas different angles of incidence result in less energy reflected back to the transducer (Figure 2.2b).

    When an ultrasound beam encounters an irregular surface, the surface will "scatter" ultrasound in all directions. This kind of interaction is called *scattering* reflection (example: muscles, liver) and results in less energy reflected back, therefore in a less echogenic (darker!) image (Figure 2.2c).

2. *Refraction.* The fraction of the ultrasound beam that is not reflected continues to travel through the tissue, but its direction is altered, or *refracted* (Figure 2.2d). The amount of refraction is related to the difference in sound velocities in the two tissues (the larger the difference, the higher the refraction) and the angle of incidence.

    A high refraction causes poor quality image and the formation of artefacts.

    - *In summary: the ideal situation to obtain a good image is always with the angle of incidence of 90 degrees and when the difference of impedance is minimal (high reflection directed to the transducer, refraction does not occur).*

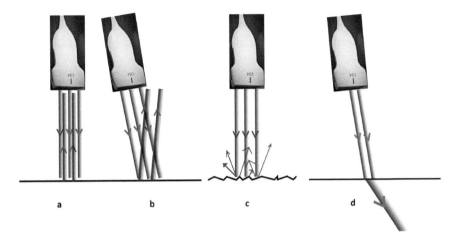

a   b   c   d

Figure 2.2 Interactions between ultrasound and tissues. a,b: reflection. c: scattering. d: refraction

3. *Attenuation.* In addition to being reflected and refracted from tissue interfaces, the ultrasound signal is attenuated travelling in uniform tissue. The attenuation in energy caused by dispersion and absorption results in less energy and a weaker signal returning to the transducer.

   • *Lower frequency signals are less attenuated. Higher frequency signals have a better spatial resolution. Therefore, to investigate a large, deep structure with ultrasound a low frequency probe will be the best (i.e., diaphragm excursion through the liver), while to investigate a small structure close to the probe (i.e., diaphragm thickness at the zone of apposition) the best choice will be a high frequency probe.*

Machine Setting

One of the frequent mistakes of beginners is to try to obtain ultrasound images without setting the machine correctly. Modern ultrasound machines have a wide range of regulations, but while some of them are easily recorded in presets and we could avoid modifying most of the time, there are four parameters that need to be well known to easily obtain the best possible image.

Frequency (or the right probe)

Ultrasound frequencies in diagnostic radiology range from 2 MHz to approximately 15 MHz.

Higher frequencies mean higher resolution. But it is important to remember that higher frequencies of ultrasound have shorter wavelengths and are absorbed/attenuated more easily. Therefore, higher frequencies are not as penetrating. This explains why high frequencies are used for the superficial body structures and low frequencies are used for those that are deeper.

Medical ultrasound transducers contain more than one operating frequency. The following frequencies are a guide to frequencies typically used for ultrasound examination:

- **2.5 MHz**: deep abdomen, obstetric, and gynaecological imaging
- **3.5 MHz**: general abdomen, obstetric, and gynaecological imaging
- **5.0 MHz**: vascular, breast, pelvic imaging
- **7.5 MHz**: breast, thyroid
- **10.0 MHz**: breast, thyroid, superficial veins, superficial masses, musculoskeletal imaging
- **15.0 MHz:** superficial structures, musculoskeletal imaging

As stated later in this book, a 2–5 MHz probe is suitable to assess diaphragm excursion across liver window, as well as 7–10 MHz is the best option to assess thickness of the diaphragm at the zone of apposition.

Depth

Depth measures are shown in cm on the side of the ultrasound monitor.

It is often best to start with a deeper view, to obtain a "macro" image and understand the anatomy of the area and then progressively reduce the depth to bring the object of interest into the middle of the screen. A short depth set could result in a loss of useful information, while a deeper assessment will produce a smaller image on our screen.

Focus

Beam focusing refers to creating a narrow point in the cross-section of the ultrasound beam called the *focal point*. It is at the focal point where the lateral resolution of the beam is also the greatest. Before the focal point is the near field or Fresnel zone, where beams converge. Distal to this focal point is the far field or Fraunhofer zone where beams diverge.

Gain/TGC

Attenuation causes a loss of ultrasound signal in the deeper field. This loss of signal results in less echogenic ("darker") images. **Gain** is a uniform amplification of the ultrasonic signal that is returning to the transducer after it travels through the tissue. So rather than brightening the monitor, the image on the screen is whitened by a uniform margin, as though the returning signal is stronger than it is, to make it easier to see. It is important to remember that gain increase simply amplifies the ultrasound signal, but it does not increase resolution (and so image quality).

A useful tool in every ultrasound machine is *time gain compensation* (TGC). TGC can compensates for the attenuation of ultrasound energy with depth (depth is synonymous with time in ultrasound!). An appropriate TGC setting allows to selectively amplify signals from structures of varying distances from the transducer, either to obtain a uniform image (Figure 2.3a) or to suppress useless farther or closer signals (Figure 2.3b).

M-mode is the time-motion display of the ultrasound wave along a chosen ultrasound line. A single scan line is emitted, received, and displayed graphically. An M-mode recording is conventionally displayed with the abscissa representing time and the ordinate distance

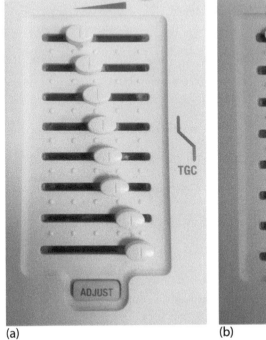
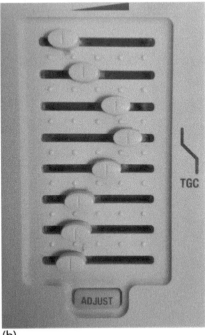

(a) (b)

Figure 2.3 (a, b) Time gain control, possible settings

Table 2.2 Steps to achieve optimal settings for B-Mode US

Steps/ settings	Remarks
Preparation	Gel, comfortable position, low lights ambient.
Gain	Signal amplitude is increased and noise is reduced with increasing gain. Adjust as low as possible to avoid overexposure. Use time gain control (TGC)/depth gain control (DGC) if necessary for compensation of strongly enhanced or diminished tissue attenuation.
Frequency	Spatial resolution is improved at the cost of depth penetration by increasing centre frequency (and inversely).
Depth penetration	No higher than required, sufficient to visualize all the structure of interest.
Focus	At the level of interest.
Further settings	Only in the case of insufficient image quality: change the preset, adjust the dynamic range, grey maps, persistence, and/or frame rate.

from the transducer, the latter derived from the time delay from echo emission to reflection and detection. All of the reflectors along this line are displayed along the time axis.

M-mode provides excellent temporal resolution and also a superior axial resolution to B-mode (i.e., the ability to discern non-contiguous structures in a vertical plane). Because of its superior dynamics and axial resolution, M-mode is the best mode for examining the timing of dynamic images (i.e., muscular contraction).

Key points

Steps to achieve optimal settings for B-Mode US are shown in Table 2.2.

o Knowing the basics of ultrasound and how your machine works will help to understand how to improve your ultrasound skills.

o Before starting, insert patient's data, set the machine correctly (right probe, right preset) gel, lower the light if possible, adopt a comfortable position.

o Once started, set depth, gain, and focus to better visualize the tissue of interest.

o TGC helps to better identify your target, especially before starting M-mode.

o Record/save images/clips to analyze, study, and compare different situations in different times (for example, changing ventilator parameters, or in case of patient worsening/improving conditions).

Resources

1. Aldrich, JE. Basic physics of ultrasound imaging. *Crit Care Med* 2007;35, No. 5 (Suppl.) S131-7

2. Tole, NM. *Basic Physics of Ultrasonic Imaging.* World Health Organization (WHO) 2005.

Part II

3

Diaphragmatic Excursion

Massimo Zambon

Diaphragmatic excursion is the perpendicular distance between the positions of the upper diaphragmatic dome at the end of expiration and at the end of inspiration. Therefore, it is related to the expansion of the thoracic cage and the ability of the diaphragm to contribute to the respiration.

First descriptions of diaphragmatic motion with ultrasound imaging dates back to the 1970s [1]. Since then, various ultrasonographic methods, such as measurement of diaphragmatic excursions by two-dimensional or M-mode and changes in diaphragm thickness during inspiration have been proposed.

The first described technique is the assessment of diaphragmatic excursion from the sub-costal window.

Technique

Either a 2–5 MHz convex probe ("abdominal") or a 3.5–5 MHz phased array ("cardiac") probe can be successfully used to assess diaphragmatic excursion.

To record the diaphragmatic motion of the right hemidiaphragm, the liver is used as a window. The probe is placed between the mid-clavicular and the anterior axillary lines, below the right costal margin, and directed medially, cranially and dorsally, so that the ultrasound beam reaches perpendicularly the posterior part of the vault of the right hemidiaphragm (Figure 3.1). The hyperechoic line adherent to the liver is due to the peritoneal and pleural lines that adhere to the diaphragm. Given the small thickness (1.5–2 mm), the distance from the probe and the image resolution, the two lines are usually not clearly distinguishable. For practical reasons, what we refer to as the diaphragm is the bright line given by the two membranes, even if this is due to the ultrasound reflection of peritoneal and pleural membranes.

DOI: 10.1201/9781003128694-5

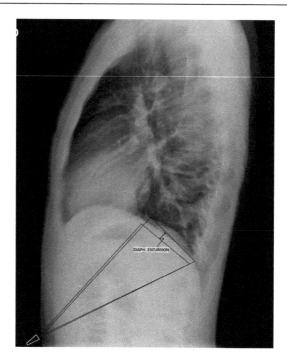

Figure 3.1 Latero-lateral chest x-ray showing the sub-costal view. Note the direction of ultrasound beam to assess the excursion of diaphragmatic dome during respiration

The inspiratory and expiratory cranio-caudal displacement of the diaphragm respectively shortens and lengthens the probe-diaphragm distance (Video 3.1).

Shifting from B-mode to M-mode, with the selected line placed perpendicularly to the upper part of the dome, the inspiratory and expiratory craniocaudal displacements appear as a bright line (hyperechoic) "waves" (Figure 3.2). To obtain a reliable measurement of the excursion, indeed the line of the M-mode must be perpendicular to the posterior part of the hemidiaphragm.

Thus, with the transducer held firmly in place, the patient is asked to engage in quiet breathing, deep breathing, or voluntary sniffing.

To measure the excursion in M-mode, the first calliper is placed at the foot of the slope of the diaphragmatic echoic line and the second calliper is placed at the apex (Figure 3.3). Considering the physiological breath-to-breath variability, at least three different recordings should be taken for each manoeuvre to calculate a mean value.

A recent imaging modality named the anatomical motion-mode (AMM) allows, through numerical image reconstruction, perfect alignment with the diaphragmatic motion. Thus, while M-Mode could overestimate diaphragmatic excursion because of uncorrected (non-perpendicular) alignment, AMM is a better option to recognize diaphragmatic dysfunction [2].

Video 3.1 2D Ultrasound (B-mode), subcostal view. Excursion of the diaphragmatic dome during respiration

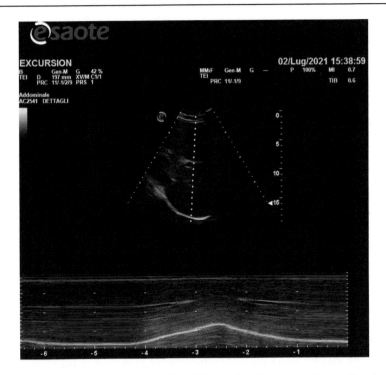

Figure 3.2 Top: B-mode (2D) assessment of the diaphragm from the sub-costal view. The diaphragm appears as a hyperechoic (white) line in the lowest part of the screen. Note the calliper for M-mode (dotted line) perpendicular to the diaphragm. Bottom: M-mode; the excursion of the diaphragm appears as a "wave", with the white line ascending (approaching the probe) during inspiration and descending during expiration

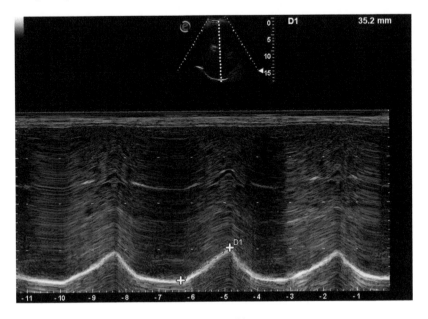

Figure 3.3 Measurement of excursion (see text for details)

On the left side, the descending lung during inspiration, bowel and stomach (gas interposition) often hide the diaphragm; therefore a more posterior approach is recommended. The dome is usually identified with the probe between the anterior and the posterior axillary lines, using the spleen window to obtain better images. The motion is recorded using M-mode US as previously described for the right side.

There are regional differences in mobility between the parts of the diaphragm that must be taken into account. During spontaneous breathing, the middle and posterior portions of the diaphragm show the greatest cranio-caudal excursion [3].

To overcome problems related to the anatomical issues, some authors have proposed alternative methods, such as:

- In B-mode: obtaining a longitudinal plane including the maximal renal bipolar length, assessing excursion as the variation of distance between the diaphragm and kidneys [4], or the craniocaudal displacement of the left branches of the portal vein (right side) and the splenic hilum or the inferior pole of the spleen (on the left) [5, 6].
- The "lung silhouette" method [7]: The transducer is placed posteriorly, at the lowest part of the lung in the scapular line. The probe orientation is longitudinal to measure the distance between the highest and lowest points of the lung silhouette during inspiration.
- The "area method": with an ultrasound machine's build-in area-calculation function, in B-mode, changes in the intra-thoracic area during respiration are calculated [8].

All these methods have been reported to allow accurate assessment of diaphragmatic excursion. Nevertheless, they are still poorly utilized and further studies are needed to assess the superiority of one method over the others.

Reference Values, Reproducibility, Learning Curves

Diaphragmatic excursion can be assessed at three time points: during quiet breathing, during deep breathing at maximal inspiration, and during voluntary sniffing.

Normal values have been previously reported for the three situations and are reported in Table 3.1

Several factors such as age, sex, anthropometric data, and position can affect diaphragmatic motion [9–12].

Table 3.1 Normal values of excursion and velocity

	Excursion (cm)		Velocity (cm/s)	
Sex	M	F	M	F
Tidal breathing	1.6	1.3	0.8	0.8
Voluntary sniff	2.0	1.7	6.7	5.2
TLC	7.9	6.4		

It has been demonstrated that diaphragm excursion measurement using the M-mode technique was a reproducible method in standing and supine patients.

The Intraclass Correlation Coefficient (ICC), inter- and intra-observer, varied between 0.88 and 0.99 [13].

Assessment of excursion with ultrasound is considered a relatively easy technique with a short learning curve. In a one-day study a combined approach was tested, consisting of a theoretical module followed by a practical training, and an accurate diaphragm displacement measurement was obtained by 91% of learners [14].

Variables other than excursion can be measured/calculated in M-mode.

- Inspiratory and expiratory time
- Diaphragm mean inspiratory velocity (cm/s): DE (in cm)/inspiratory time (in seconds)
- Expiratory velocity: exp excursion/expiratory time

The clinical usefulness of these variables should be defined with further research, and some of them will be discussed further in this book.

Usefulness

In spontaneously breathing patients, a diaphragmatic dysfunction or fatigue causes a reduced excursion. A paralyzed diaphragm can have no movement or a negative wave ("paradoxical"), due to the passive upside excursion related to the compensatory contraction of the contralateral hemidiaphragm (in case of unilateral paralysis) or the accessory respiratory muscles (Figure 3.4). Indeed, on the paralyzed side a paradoxical motion can be observed at

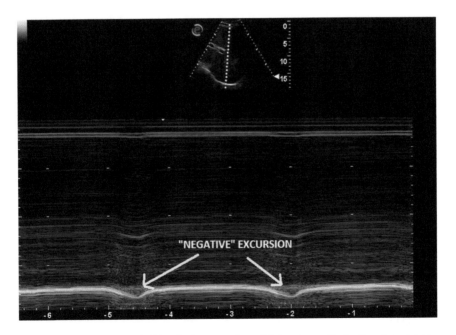

Figure 3.4 M-mode ultrasound of the diaphragm, sub-costal view, in a patient with unilateral right diaphragmatic paralysis and paradoxical movement

the beginning of the inspiration. This is due to the balance between the decrease in pleural pressure because of the force generated by the intact hemidiaphragm and the inspiratory accessory muscles, which induces a caudal displacement [15].

Importantly, it can be useful to study the diaphragmatic displacements in the supine position. Indeed, in this position the abdominal visceral mass increases the diaphragmatic work, and it has been reported that the supine position increased paradoxical movement and decreased the compensatory active expiration by the anterior abdominal wall [16]. This may mask the paralysis.

In patients suffering from hemidiaphragm paralysis, the measurement of the excursions on the healthy side can be informative. Indeed, large excursions of the normal side are more frequently observed during quiet breathing in relation to a compensatory mechanism. These aspects are further discussed in Chapter 5.

Excursion on Ventilated Patients

Diaphragmatic excursion is influenced by mechanical ventilation. In mechanically ventilated patients, the usefulness and interpretation of US measurements is related to ventilator settings.

Under controlled mechanical ventilation (CMV), the patient respiratory workload is null, and the diaphragmatic excursion is related to the tidal volumes. Therefore, in CMV excursion cannot give any information about (residual) diaphragmatic function.

During assisted mechanical ventilation (namely pressure support ventilation, PSV), the diaphragmatic excursion measured with ultrasound is the result of the sum of the patient's effort and pressure support given by the ventilator. However, since diaphragmatic excursion is related to tidal volumes [4, 17], compliance of the respiratory system plays an important role in diaphragmatic excursion. In fact, in a patient with low respiratory system compliance, the same pressure support added to the same patient's effort will result in a low tidal volume, causing a minor displacement of the diaphragm. On the other side, a respiratory system with higher compliance will show a higher tidal volume and a larger diaphragmatic excursion [18].

The expected effect of Positive End Expiratory Pressure (PEEP) or Continuous Positive Airways Pressure (CPAP during invasive and non-invasive ventilation is to increase functional residual capacity (FRC), maintaining alveolar recruitment; the corresponding increase in lung volumes lowers diaphragmatic dome [19]. This effect can result in a decreased diaphragmatic excursion, not related to diaphragmatic dysfunction but to a caudal displacement of diaphragmatic dome at the end of expiration.

Finally, patient's position should be carefully considered during diaphragmatic excursion measurements with ultrasonography. Trans-diaphragmatic pressure is the result of the difference between abdominal and thoracic pressures: diaphragmatic muscular force acts against abdominal pressure, and the magnitude of this force is higher in the supine position than in semi-recumbent or seated position. This effect is stronger in obese patients and in patients with intra-abdominal hypertension [20]. Hence, repeated measures should be taken in the same position to avoid pitfalls in evaluation of diaphragmatic function over time in the same patient.

Key points

- o *The excursions of the two hemidiaphragms during respiration can be measured using two-dimensional or (better) M-mode ultrasonography, during quiet breathing, voluntary sniffing, and deep inspiration.*
- o *Excursion is related to diaphragmatic function in spontaneously breathing patients.*
- o *A paralyzed diaphragm can show paradoxical movement during breathing.*
- o *Factors such as position and intra-abdominal pressure influences excursion.*
- o *During controlled mechanical ventilation, excursion is solely related to the tidal volumes. In assisted modes, excursion is related to a combination of ventilator and muscular workload.*

References

1. Haber K, Asher M, Freimanis AK. Echographic evaluation of diaphragmatic motion in intra-abdominal diseases. *Radiology* 1975;114:141–4.

2. Pasero D, Koeltz A, Placido R, Fontes Lima M, Haun O, Rienzo M, Marrache D, Pirracchio R, Safran D, Cholley B. Improving ultrasonic measurement of diaphragmatic excursion after cardiac surgery using the anatomical M-mode: a randomized crossover study. *Intensive Care Med* 2015 Apr;41(4):650–6.

3. Harris RS, Giovannetti M, Kim BK. Normal ventilatory movement of the right hemidiaphragm studied by ultrasonography and pneumotachography. *Radiology* 1983;146(1):141–4.

4. Houston JG, Angus RM, Cowan MD, McMillan NC, Thomson NC. Ultrasound assessment of normal hemidiaphragmatic movement: relation to inspiratory volume. *Thorax* 1994;49:500–3.

5. Toledo NS, Kodaira SK, Massarollo PC, Pereira OI, Mies S. Right hemidiaphragmatic mobility: assessment with US measurement of craniocaudal displacement of left branches of portal vein. *Radiology* 2003;228:389–94.

6. Toledo NS, Kodaira SK, Massarollo PC, Pereira OI, Dalmas JC, Cerri GG, Buchpiguel CA. Left hemidiaphragmatic mobility: assessment with ultrasonographic measurement of the craniocaudal displacement of the splenic hilum and the inferior pole of the spleen. *J Ultrasound Med* 2006;25:41–9.

7. Scheibe N, Sosnowski N, Pinkhasik A, Vonderbank S, Bastian A. Sonographic evaluation of diaphragmatic dysfunction in COPD patients. *Int J Chron Obstruct Pulmon Dis* 2015;10:1925–30.

8. Skaarup SH, Løkke A, Laursen CB. The area method: a new method for ultrasound assessment of diaphragmatic movement. *Crit Ultrasound J* 2018;10:15.

9. Boussuges A, Brégeon F, Blanc P, Gil JM, Poirette L. Characteristics of the paralysed diaphragm studied by M-mode ultrasonography. *Clin Physiol Funct Imaging* 2019;39:143–9.

10. Scarlata S, Mancini D, Laudisio A, Benigni A, Antonelli Incalzi R. Reproducibility and clinical correlates of supine diaphragmatic motion measured by M-mode ultrasonography in healthy volunteers. *Respiration* 2018;96:259–66.

11. Kantarci F, Mihmanli I, Demirel MK, Harmanci K, Akman C, Aydogan F, Mihmanli A, Uysal O. Normal diaphragmatic motion and the effects of body composition: determination with M-mode sonography. *J Ultrasound Med* 2004;23:255–60.

12. Spiesshoefer J, Herkenrath S, Henke C, Langenbruch L, Schneppe M, Randerath W, Young P, Brix T, Boentert M. Evaluation of respiratory muscle strength and diaphragm ultrasound: normative values, theoretical considerations, and practical recommendations. *Respiration* 2020;99(5):369–81.

13. Zambon M, Greco M, Bocchino S, Cabrini L, Beccaria PF, Zangrillo A. Assessment of diaphragmatic dysfunction in the critically ill patient with ultrasound: a systematic review. *Intensive Care Med* 2017 Jan;43(1):29–38. doi: 10.1007/s00134-016-4524-z. Epub 2016 Sep 12. PMID: 27620292.

14. Garofalo E, Bruni A, Pelaia C, Landoni G, Zangrillo A, Antonelli M, Conti G, Biasucci DG, Mercurio G, Cortegiani A, Giarratano A, Vetrugno L, Bove T, Forfori F, Corradi F, Vaschetto R, Cammarota G, Astuto M, Murabito P, Bellini V, Zambon M, Longhini F, Navalesi P, Bignami E. Comparisons of two diaphragm ultrasound-teaching programs: a multicenter randomized controlled educational study. *Ultrasound J* 2019 Oct 3;11(1):21.

15. Gottesman E, McCool FD. Ultrasound evaluation of the paralyzed diaphragm. *Am J Respir Crit Care Med* 1997;155:1570–4.

16. Scillia P, Cappello M, De Troyer A. Determinants of diaphragm motion in unilateral diaphragmatic paralysis. *J Appl Physiol* 2004; 96: 96–100.

17. Cohen E, Mier A, Heywood P, Murphy K, Boultbee J, Guz A. Excursion-volume relation of the right hemidiaphragm measured by ultrasonography and respiratory airflow measurements. *Thorax* 1994;49:885–9.

18. Zambon M, Cabrini L, Beccaria P, Zangrillo A, Colombo S. Ultrasound in critically ill patients: focus on diaphragm. *Intensive Care Med* 2013;39:986

19. Beaumont M, Lejeune D, Marotte H, Harf A, Lofaso F. Effects of chest wall counterpressures on lung mechanics under high levels of CPAP in humans. *J Appl Physiol* 1997;83:591–8.

20. Pelosi P, Luecke T, Rocco PR. Chest wall mechanics and abdominal pressure during general anaesthesia in normal and obese individuals and in acute lung injury. *Curr Opin Crit Care* 2011;17:72–9.

4

Diaphragmatic Thickness and Thickening

Massimo Zambon

Thickness and thickening of the diaphragm can be assessed with ultrasound at the zone of apposition (ZOA). The ZOA extends from the diaphragm's caudal insertion near the costal margin, to the costophrenic angle, where the fibres break away from the rib cage to form the free diaphragmatic dome. While the dome of the diaphragm corresponds to the central tendon, the majority of the muscular portion of the diaphragm lies directly in the ZOA (*see Chapter 2*).

The area of apposition of diaphragm to rib cage makes up a substantial but variable fraction of the total surface area of the rib cage. During quiet breathing in the upright posture, it represents one fourth to one third of the total surface area of the rib cage. The cephalic extreme begins approximately below the eighth intercostal space and extends to the eleventh.

In this region the diaphragm is a relatively superficial structure parallelly oriented with the skin surface. Therefore, its assessment with ultrasound is favoured because of:

A. Proximity to the probe.
B. The ultrasound beam is perpendicular to the diaphragm, giving the best results in terms of image resolution (see Chapter 1).
C. Echogenicity of pleural and peritoneum layers, that *facilitates* the identification of the diaphragm.

The first report of the technique and its validation dates more than 30 years ago [1]. In a study published in 1989, Wait and co-workers described the measurement of diaphragm thickness with ultrasound at the zone of apposition, validating the method in situ at necropsy, verifying

DOI: 10.1201/9781003128694-6

the measurements of the same segment by ruler. They found a very good correlation between anatomic measurements and ultrasound assessment. Furthermore, they repeated the study in ten healthy volunteers, studying diaphragmatic function in terms of variations of thickness and correlation with tidal volumes. Recently, many authors studied and validated ultrasound assessment of diaphragm thickness, mainly in the setting of critical care and pneumology [2–5].

Usefulness

Ultrasound is the method of choice to measure thickness of the diaphragm, and therefore to detect atrophy and to monitor its time-course. Diaphragmatic atrophy may be present in different pathologic entities, such as disuse atrophy caused by mechanical ventilation, even after relatively short periods of ventilation [6–10]. Atrophy and dysfunction of the muscle implies a limited force generation and patients are often difficult to wean from mechanical ventilation. In a systematic review, DU was found successfully applied in the critically ill patients in four different settings [11]:

1. To assess the progression of atrophy in ICU mechanically ventilated patients.
2. To diagnose dysfunction or paralysis. DD diagnosed with ultrasound was found in about 30% of mechanically ventilated patients without history of diaphragmatic or neuromuscular disease.
3. To predict weaning success/failure from mechanical ventilation. Thickening fraction measurements performed during a spontaneous breathing trial in intubated patients has shown good performance as weaning index.
4. To assess patient respiratory workload in assisted mechanical ventilation. When compared to invasive techniques such as diaphragm and oesophagal time–pressure product (PTPdi and PTPes), the thickening fraction has shown significant correlation, thus emerging as a new non-invasive tool to monitor a previously neglected respiratory parameter.

Furthermore, in non-critical care setting the monitoring of ongoing atrophy and reduced contractility have been applied for a wide spectrum of pathological entities involving respiratory muscles such as neuromuscular diseases, paralysis, COPD, asthma, and other respiratory disorders (see Chapters 2 and 10).

How to Measure Thickness

The diaphragm at the ZOA is a very thin (1.5–2.5 mm), superficial structure. Since the resolution is directly correlated with ultrasound frequency, and frequency is inversely correlated with ultrasound attenuation, a high frequency (usually 7–15 MHz) linear probe is essential to visualize the diaphragm. The resolution needed is at least 0.1 mm to correctly measure the thickness.

The probe is placed between the eighth and tenth intercostal space in the midaxillary or anteroaxillary line and the ultrasound beam is directed perpendicular to the rib cage (Figure 4.1). The inferior border of the costophrenic sinus can be identified as the zone of transition from the artefactual representation of normal lung (the lung sliding, Video 4.1)

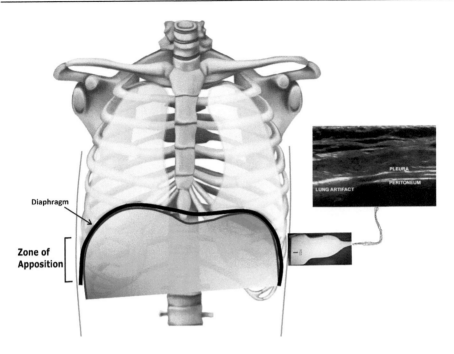

Figure 4.1 Assessment of the diaphragm at the zone of apposition

Video 4.1 2D (B-mode) visualization of the diaphragm at the ZOA. Note the lung sliding coming from the right side of the image, hiding the diaphragm.

to the visualization of liver (right side) or bowel/spleen (left side). The ZOA is 1–3 cm below the costophrenic sinus. Below skin surface and subcutaneous tissue, two parallel echogenic layers are identified at a depth of 2–3 cm: the nearest line is the parietal pleura, the deepest is the peritoneum just superficial to the liver or the spleen. These two membranes adhere to the diaphragm; therefore, the less echogenic structure in between the two lines is the muscle (Figure 4.2).

To avoid over-estimation of thickness, the ultrasound beam must reach the diaphragm with an angle of 90°. The diaphragm thickness can be measured in B-mode, or better in M-mode, as the distance between the outer edges of the echogenic lines at end-expiration.

While the right hemidiaphragm is always easily accessible, assessment of the left hemidiaphragm is sometimes difficult to obtain [5, 10].

How to Measure Thickening

The contraction of the diaphragm, just like the one of every other muscle, causes the shortening and thickening of fibres. Therefore, measuring thickness variation with respiratory activity allows to detect diaphragmatic activity as well.

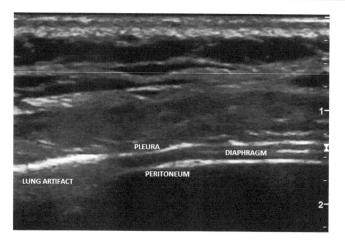

Figure 4.2 B-mode visualization of the diaphragm at the ZOA

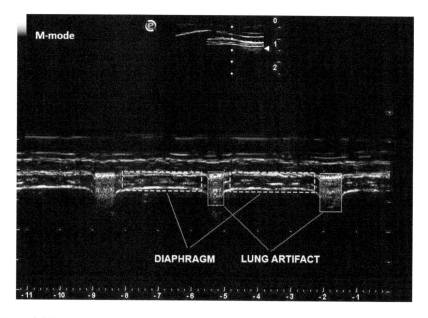

Figure 4.3 M-mode: the diaphragm is hidden by the lung sliding during inspiration

The technique is the same used to measure thickness. It is important to detect the end of the inspiratory act (maximal contraction, higher value of thickness) and the end of expiratory act (relaxed diaphragm, lowest value of thickness). The measurement can be done during normal breathing, therefore measuring thickening "at rest", or asking the patient to perform a maximal inspiratory effort, therefore measuring thickening at total lung capacity (TLC). The latter is the best choice to assess diaphragm capacity of contraction but requires a perfectly cooperative patient.

In M-mode, the lowest possible scan velocity should be selected, to better visualize the two echogenic lines. During deep breathing, the overlapped lung sliding artefact tends to erase the diaphragm (Figure 4.3, Video 4.1); therefore, the probe must be replaced slightly caudal,

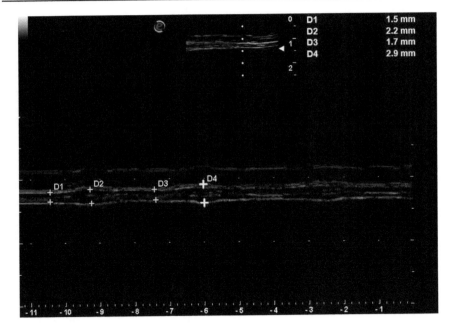

Figure 4.4 M-mode: diaphragm thickening during normal breathing

just 1–2 cm lower than the lowest point reached by lung sliding. Furthermore, we suggest decreasing the gain at the lowest level, which allows to visualize the pleural and peritoneal lines avoiding unnecessary noise due to other echogenic structures (Figure 4.4).

At least three measurements should be taken, and the values should be averaged.

Change in diaphragm thickness with respiratory movement can be expressed as a percentage called the thickening fraction of the diaphragm (TFdi):*

$$TFdi = (TEI - TEE) / TEE\%$$

(TEI: thickening at end inspiration, or maximal thickening; TEE: thickening at end expiration measured when the diaphragm is relaxed.)

Diaphragm thickening during inspiration reflects diaphragm shortening and is somewhat analogous to an "ejection fraction" of the heart. In spontaneously breathing cooperative patients, it must be specified if thickening fraction is assessed obtaining a deep breath like in spirometry tests. Hence, TEI is the thickening at total lung capacity (TLC), while TEE is the thickening at functional residual capacity (FRC) (Figure 4.5).

The greater the thickening, the higher is the inspiratory effort. On the other side, a "fatigued" diaphragm may be not able to thicken sufficiently, and a reduced thickening in a tachypnoeic patient may be a sign of diaphragmatic dysfunction. Thickening of the diaphragm has been tested as an index of respiratory workload both in spontaneous breathing [1–3] and in mechanically non-invasive and invasively ventilated patients [12–14]. TF has a linear correlation with Tidal Volume in spontaneous breathing subjects, whereas in mechanically ventilated patients thickening is related to the patient's workload and is "suppressed" by the

---

*The thickening fraction has been described in literature also as Δtdi% (percent change in tdi between end expiration and end inspiration), delta t(di), DTF (diaphragmatic thickness fraction), and other acronyms.

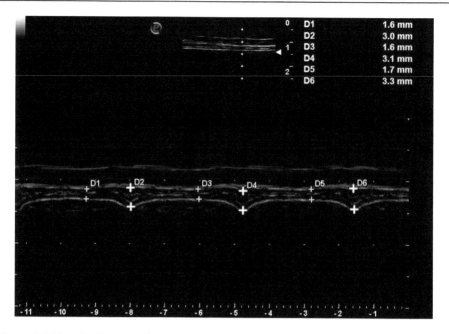

0	D1	1.6 mm
	D2	3.0 mm
1	D3	1.6 mm
	D4	3.1 mm
2	D5	1.7 mm
	D6	3.3 mm

Figure 4.5 M-mode: thickening of the diaphragm during a deep breath at functional residual capacity

ventilator support. As expected, in assisted mechanical ventilation modes, thickening of the diaphragm increases with the decrease of ventilator support while in controlled modes thickening tends towards zero as the respiratory muscles become inactive.

Reference Values

Several publications have reported reference values of diaphragm thickness and thickening. There is a quite high variability in the reference values reported in literature, likely due to technical issues. Notably, some authors recommend measuring the distance between the inner edges of the two echogenic lines, while others include the pleural and peritoneal lines in the measurements, thus increasing the measured thickness. In a recent consensus of experts (*Exodus, submitted*), a recommendation was stated to limit the measurement to the less echogenic space internal to the echogenic lines. This clarification is important in terms of reproducibility, as two different ways of measurement can result in a difference as high as 20%.

In healthy, spontaneously breathing subjects, the normal thickness of the diaphragm at the ZOA ranges from 1.7 ± 0.3 mm while relaxing, to 3–4 mm when breath holding at total lung capacity (TLC). These values vary according to sex: in a large observational study in young healthy subjects, diaphragm thickness was found to be an average of 1.3 ± 0.3 mm in women, 1.8 ± 0.4 mm in men. Furthermore, it varies significantly with BMI and thorax circumference [15]. There is no evidence of variation with age.

Thickening fraction in healthy subjects spontaneously breathing at rest is 20–40% and can increase to 200% while breathing at TLC. Interestingly, some reports in patients with diaphragm paralysis report TF values <0 (negative) [4]. This could be due to a sort of "stretching" mechanism on diaphragmatic fibres caused by compensation activity of accessory respiratory muscles.

Meaning of Reduced/Increased

Reproducibility

Ultrasound performed at zone of apposition has high reproducibility and accuracy, with intraclass correlation coefficients ranging from 0.876 to 0.999 for intra-observer agreement and from 0.56 to 0.989 for interobserver agreement [11, 16].

Learning Curve

There are no sufficient data to define how much time and work is necessary to build solid expertise in diaphragm ultrasound.

In adult patients, the training of ultrasound operators to identify the diaphragm and measure its thickness was reported to take three to five sessions lasting 10–15 min each [17].

A recent study hypothesized that combining a video tutorial and practical session could be sufficient to obtain sufficient skills [18]. As possible bias, the study was conducted only in healthy subjects, and the assessment of diaphragm thickness and thickening in critically ill, mechanically ventilated patients is often more difficult because of some oedema, non-cooperative patients, and other misleading factors.

Even if reported learning curves are quite short, indicating ultrasound at the ZOA an "easy to perform" tool, some issues should be considered. First, the best resolution (that corresponds to the smallest measurable distance) of most machines is 0.1 mm, which means about 5–7% of the thickness measured; second, technical difficulties with some patients (i.e., obese patients) should be expected; third, asymmetry between the two hemidiaphragms is often present but it is not always possible to assess the left hemidiaphragm. Therefore, small operator-dependent variations could influence the measurement and consistency should be aimed at when repeated measures are necessary (i.e., same operator, marked anatomic site of measurement, same machine setting, etc.).

Key points

o Right side is usually better visualized than left side probably because of air (colon) under the diaphragm on the left side, while on the right side the liver creates an optimal acoustic window.

o To better identify the diaphragm in M-mode, it is useful to play with the TGC setting to obtain a darker image above and under the two lines and slightly brighten in the depth of the muscle.

o To quickly identify the right place to make the measurements, it is better to start from the bottom of the lung sliding.

o Record several breathing cycles and consider the widest, to avoid a possible under estimation of TF caused by intrinsic respiratory variability.

o Take more than one measurement (usually 3) to increase reproducibility.

References

1. Wait JL, Nahormek PA, Yost WT, Rochester DP. Diaphragmatic thickness lung volume relationship invivo. *J Appl Physiol* 1989;67:1560–8.

2. Cohn D, Benditt JO, Eveloff S, McCool FD. Diaphragm thickening during inspiration. *J Appl Physiol* 1997;83(1):291–6.

3. Ueki J, De Bruin PF, Pride NB. In vivo assessment of diaphragm contraction by ultrasound in normal subjects. *Thorax* 1995;50:1157–61.

4. Gottesman E, McCool FD. Ultrasound evaluation of the paralyzed diaphragm. *Am J Respir Crit Care Med* 1997;155:1570–4.

5. Goligher EC, Laghi F, Detsky ME, Farias P, Murray A, Brace D, Brochard LJ, Bolz SS, Rubenfeld GD, Kavanagh BP, Ferguson ND. Measuring diaphragm thickness with ultrasound in mechanically ventilated patients: feasibility, reproducibility and validity *Intensive Care Med* 2015;41:734.

6. Levine S, Nguyen T, Taylor N, Friscia ME, Budak MT, Rothenberg P, Zhu J, Sachdeva R, Sonnad S, Kaiser LR, Rubinstein NA, Powers SK, Shrager JB. Rapid disuse atrophy of diaphragm fibers in mechanically ventilated humans. *N Engl J Med* 2008 Mar 27;358(13):1327–35.

7. Vivier ERA, Doroszewski F, Roselli S, Pommier C, Carteaux G, Dessap AM. Atrophy of diaphragm and pectoralis muscles in critically ill patients. *Anesthesiology* 2019;131:569–79.

8. Dubé BP, Dres M, Mayaux J, Demiri S, Similowski T, Demoule A. Ultrasound evaluation of diaphragm function in mechanically ventilated patients: comparison to phrenic stimulation and prognostic implications. *Thorax* 2017;72:811–18.

9. Goligher EC, Dres M, Fan E, Rubenfeld GD, Scales DC, Herridge MS, Vorona S, Sklar MC, Rittayamai N, Lanys A, Murray A, Brace D, Urrea C, Reid WD, Tomlinson G, Slutsky AS, Kavanagh BP, Brochard LJ, Ferguson ND. Mechanical ventilation-induced diaphragm atrophy strongly impacts clinical outcomes. *Am J Respir Crit Care Med* 2018;197:204–13.

10. Zambon M, Beccaria P, Matsuno J, Gemma M, Frati E, Colombo S, Cabrini L, Landoni G, Zangrillo A. Mechanical ventilation and diaphragmatic atrophy in critically ill patients: an ultrasound study. *Crit Care Med* 2016 Jul;44(7):1347–52.

11. Zambon M, Greco M, Bocchino S, Cabrini L, Beccaria PF, Zangrillo A. Assessment of diaphragmatic dysfunction in the critically ill patient with ultrasound: a systematic review. *Intensive Care Med* 2017;43:29–38.

12. Vivier E, Mekontso Dessap A, Dimassi S, Vargas F, Lyazidi A, Thille AW, Brochard L. Diaphragm ultrasonography to estimate the work of breathing during non-invasive ventilation. *Intensive Care Med* 2012;38:796–803.

13. Umbrello M, Formenti P, Longhi D, Galimberti A, Piva I, Pezzi A, Mistraletti G, Marini JJ, Iapichino G. Diaphragm ultrasound as indicator of respiratory effort in critically ill patients undergoing assisted mechanical ventilation: a pilot clinical study. *Crit Care* 2015;19:161.

14. Goligher EC, Laghi F, Detsky ME, et al. Measuring diaphragm thickness with ultrasound in mechanically ventilated patients: feasibility, reproducibility and validity. *Intensive Care Med* 2015;41:642–9.

15. Carrillo-Esper R, Perez-Calatayud AA, Arch-Tirado E, Diaz-Carrillo MA, Garrido-Aguirre E, Tapia-Velazco R, Pena-Perez CA, Espinoza-de Los Monteros I, Meza-Marquez JM, Flores-Rivera OI, Zepeda-Mendoza AD, de la Torre-Leon T. Standardization of sonographic diaphragm thickness evaluations in healthy volunteers. *Respir Care* 2016;61:920–4.

16. Santana PV, Cárdenas LZ, Albuquerque ALP, Carvalho CRR, Caruso PJ. Diaphragmatic ultrasound: a review of its methodological aspects and clinical uses. *Bras Pneumol* 2020;46(6):e2020006.

17. Dinino E, Gartman EJ, Sethi JM et al. Diaphragm ultrasound as a predictor of successful extubation from mechanical ventilation. *Thorax* 2014;69:431–5.

18. Garofalo E, Bruni A, Pelaia C, Landoni G, Zangrillo A, Antonelli M, Conti G, Biasucci DG, Mercurio G, Cortegiani A, Giarratano A, Vetrugno L, Bove T, Forfori F, Corradi F, Vaschetto R, Cammarota G, Astuto M, Murabito P, Bellini V, Zambon M, Longhini F, Navalesi P, Bignami E. Comparisons of two diaphragm ultrasound-teaching programs: a multicenter randomized controlled educational study. *Ultrasound J* 2019 Oct 3;11(1):21.

Part III

Applications of Diaphragm Ultrasound

5

Diaphragm Ultrasound in Respiratory Disorders and Diaphragm Paralysis

Pauliane Vieira Santana, Leticia Zumpano Cardenas, and Andre Luis Pereira de Albuquerque

DOI: 10.1201/9781003128694-8

Diaphragm Ultrasound in Respiratory Disorders and Diaphragm Paralysis

Dyspnea and exercise intolerance are common in chronic respiratory diseases contributing to poor quality of life (1). Different pathophysiological mechanisms underlie exertional dyspnea in chronic respiratory diseases, but it is usually linked to increased neural drive to inspiratory muscles, eliciting an increased inspiratory muscle effort with a blunted tidal volume (TV) expansion reflecting a neuromechanical dissociation (NMD) (2).

It is therefore relevant to understand the respiratory muscle function, particularly diaphragm function, in chronic respiratory diseases.

Diaphragm ultrasound (DUS) may disclose various aspects of diaphragm function and structure (3) with a non-invasive and real-time method:

- Diaphragmatic thickness and length may assess muscle structure.
- Diaphragmatic mobility and maximum thickening may assess function.
- Diaphragmatic thickening fraction may assess activity (effort and contractility).
- Diaphragmatic thickening as a fraction of maximum thickening may assess force-reserve.

COPD

Rationale for Diaphragmatic Dysfunction in COPD

COPD is a progressive inflammatory disease characterized by increased airway resistance and airflow limitation.

Airflow limitation decreases dynamic lung compliance and increases the intrinsic PEEP overloading inspiratory muscles and diaphragmatic work of breathing. Exercise exacerbates these effects due to dynamic hyperinflation (1, 4) that intensifies critical dynamic constraints:

- There is a critical reduction of inspiratory reserve volume (IRV), blunting VT expansion, close to TLC (upper non-linear respiratory pressure–volume relationship).
- Diaphragm works on a mechanical disadvantage at high values of FRC (diaphragmatic suboptimal length due to the flattening of its curvature and reduced apposition to the chest wall), increasing diaphragm workload and reducing force-generating capacity (5, 6).
- Also, diaphragmatic dysfunction may occur in COPD because of cellular mechanisms such as oxidative stress (7), remodelling with reduced myosin filaments (8, 9).

Diaphragmatic Mobility in COPD

Dos Santos Yamaguti et al. (10) assessed the diaphragm mobility and its relationship with pulmonary function, and respiratory muscle strength in COPD patients ($n = 54$) and healthy subjects ($n = 20$). They found that, compared to controls, COPD patients had lower diaphragmatic mobility, which was mainly associated with air trapping, but was not influenced by inspiratory strength or pulmonary hyperinflation.

Scheibe et al. (11) compared two methods to visualize and measure the diaphragmatic mobility in COPD ($n = 60$) and healthy subjects ($n = 20$). Their method revealed reliable results and showed that compared to controls, COPD patients had lower diaphragmatic mobility that was strongly correlated with FEV_1.

Reduced Diaphragmatic Mobility in COPD – Clinical Relevance

Paulin et al. (12) assessed the diaphragm mobility and its relationship with exercise tolerance and dyspnea in COPD patients ($n = 50$) in comparison with healthy subjects ($n = 20$). They found that COPD patients had decreased diaphragmatic mobility that was correlated positively with distance covered on the 6-min walk test, but negatively with exertional dyspnea.

Recently, Shiraishi et al. (13) assessed the correlation of diaphragmatic excursions (DE) with exercise tolerance and dynamic lung hyperinflation in COPD patients ($n = 20$), in comparison with matched controls ($n = 20$). They found that, compared to controls, COPD patients presented significantly lower maximal DE, which was related to exercise intolerance (decreased exercise capacity and increased dyspnea) and dynamic lung hyperinflation.

Diaphragmatic Thickness in COPD

Baria et al. (14) investigated whether DUS (diaphragm thickness at quiet end-expiration – Tdi, and thickening ratio – TR) could provide a simple and safe mean to assess for coexisting neuromuscular respiratory weakness in COPD patients. They measured Tdi and TR in COPD patients ($n = 50$) and compared with a database of healthy controls ($n = 150$). COPD and controls presented similar values for Tdi and TR.

Smargiassi et al. (15) investigated the relationships between diaphragmatic thickness – TD, at different lung volumes, respiratory function, and body composition in COPD patients ($n = 32$). They found that TD at different lung volumes, mainly the Tdi, were related to free fat mass (FFM) and that diaphragmatic thickening was inversely related to hyperinflation, arguing about the DUS usefulness to assess lung hyperinflation and FFM loss in COPD.

Okura et al. (16) measured diaphragmatic thickness (TD) and thickening in COPD ($n = 38$) comparing it to healthy younger (22 ± 1 years; $n = 15$) and healthy older adults (72 ± 5 years; $n = 15$) to assess the influence of ageing and/or COPD on diaphragm function. TD was measured at total lung capacity (TD_{TLC}), at functional residual capacity (TD_{FRC}), and residual volume (TD_{RV}), and the change ratio was calculated from TD_{RV} to TD_{TLC} ($\Delta Tdi\,\%$). They showed that TD_{TLC} and the $\Delta Tdi\%$ were lower in COPD patients compared to healthy adults. Age did not influence diaphragm thickness or thickening.

Altered Diaphragmatic Thickness in COPD – Clinical Relevance

Rittayamai et al. (17) investigated the diaphragmatic function (activity, function, and force reserve) in COPD patients ($n = 80$) compared to healthy controls ($n = 20$) to assess whether there was impairment of diaphragmatic function in COPD, and if so, if diaphragmatic dysfunction of COPD would be related to lung volumes and COPD exacerbation. They found that, when compared to controls, COPD patients had greater tidal thickening fraction of the diaphragm, but lower diaphragmatic maximal thickening fraction and force reserve ratio, reflecting poorer diaphragm function, which was related with COPD severity (GOLD stage), inspiratory capacity, and the BODE index. Further, COPD patients who developed exacerbation during the following two years had decreased force reserve.

Diaphragmatic Function Assessed by DUS and Interventions

Corbellini et al. (18) assessed diaphragmatic mobility in moderate to severe COPD patients ($n = 52$) who underwent pulmonary rehabilitation (PR) and healthy subjects ($n = 16$). They investigated whether diaphragmatic mobility was related with COPD severity and could be improved by PR. Interestingly, they found that when compared with controls, quiet breathing diaphragmatic mobility was higher in COPD, while deep breathing diaphragmatic mobility was lower. The diaphragmatic mobility was correlated with FEV_1. Diaphragmatic mobility loss improved after in-patient PR.

Crimi et al. (19) evaluated changes in diaphragmatic mobility and thickness after pulmonary rehabilitation (PR) in COPD patients ($n = 25$) and assessed its correlation with PR outcomes. They found that PR improved diaphragmatic mobility and increased the length of the diaphragmatic zone of apposition (Lzapp). The improvement of Lzapp after PR in COPD significantly correlated with improvement in the 6-minute walking distance and CAT scores, revealing that DUS accurately identified COPD patients who improved after PR.

Diaphragm Function and Acute Exacerbations of COPD (AECOPD) – Thickness

Antenora et al. (20) investigated the prevalence of diaphragmatic dysfunction (DD) and its impact on the outcomes (non-invasive mechanical ventilation (NIV) failure, length of hospital stay and mortality) of severe AECOPD patients ($n = 41$) admitted to intensive care unit – ICU. DUS was performed on admission before starting NIV, and a change in diaphragmatic thickness (ΔTdi) less than 20% during spontaneous breathing defined diaphragmatic dysfunction (DD+). They found a prevalence of 24.3% of DD+ which was associated with steroid use and poorer outcomes (NIV failure, longer ICU stay, prolonged Mechanical Ventilation (MV), need for tracheostomy, and higher ICU mortality). This study suggested that assessment of DD in AECOPD patients might identify those at major risk of adverse outcomes.

This previous study (20) was extended by the authors to investigate the impact of diaphragmatic dysfunction (DD) on outcomes of AECOPD patients ($n = 75$) admitted to the ICU (21). Again, DD was associated with poorer clinical outcomes (higher risk for NIV failure; higher ICU, in-hospital, and 90-day mortality rates; prolonged MV; higher tracheostomy rate; and longer ICU stay).

Diaphragm Function and AECOPD – Excursion

Abbas et al. (22) performed DUS on a sample of ready-to-wean AECOPD patients ($n = 50$), during a T-tube spontaneous breathing trial. They investigated whether diaphragmatic-rapid shallow breathing index (D-RSBI = the ratio between respiratory rate (RR) and the diaphragmatic displacement = DD) could predict the weaning outcome in comparison with the traditional RSBI (RR/VT). They found that D-RSBI was superior (AUC = 0.97) to the RSBI (AUC = 0.67) in predicting weaning outcome in AECOPD patients.

Lim et al. (23) investigated the changes in diaphragmatic function (diaphragmatic excursion and thickening fraction – TF) during AECOPD ($n = 10$), performed within 72 hours after exacerbation and after symptoms' improvement. They found that TF (but not the diaphragmatic excursion) showed a significant increase from the initial to the follow-up. However, the change in diaphragmatic excursion (from the stable to the exacerbation period) correlated positively with the time to the next exacerbation and negatively with the recovery time from the exacerbation.

Similarly, Cammarota et al. (24) investigated the diaphragmatic function (excursion, thickness, and TF) during AECOPD subjects ($n = 21$) admitted to the emergency department. They evaluated the feasibility of performing DUS before starting NIV (T0), after the first (T1) and second hour (T2) of treatment, and assessed whether DUS findings could predict early NIV failure. They found that diaphragmatic excursion (but not Tdi and TF) was greater in NIV successes than in NIV failures (at all times), and so diaphragmatic excursion could predict NIV failure during AECOPD.

Figure 5.1 illustrates the findings of DUS in a AECOPD patient.

Table 5.1 illustrates the main findings of DUS in COPD and its possible clinical relevance.

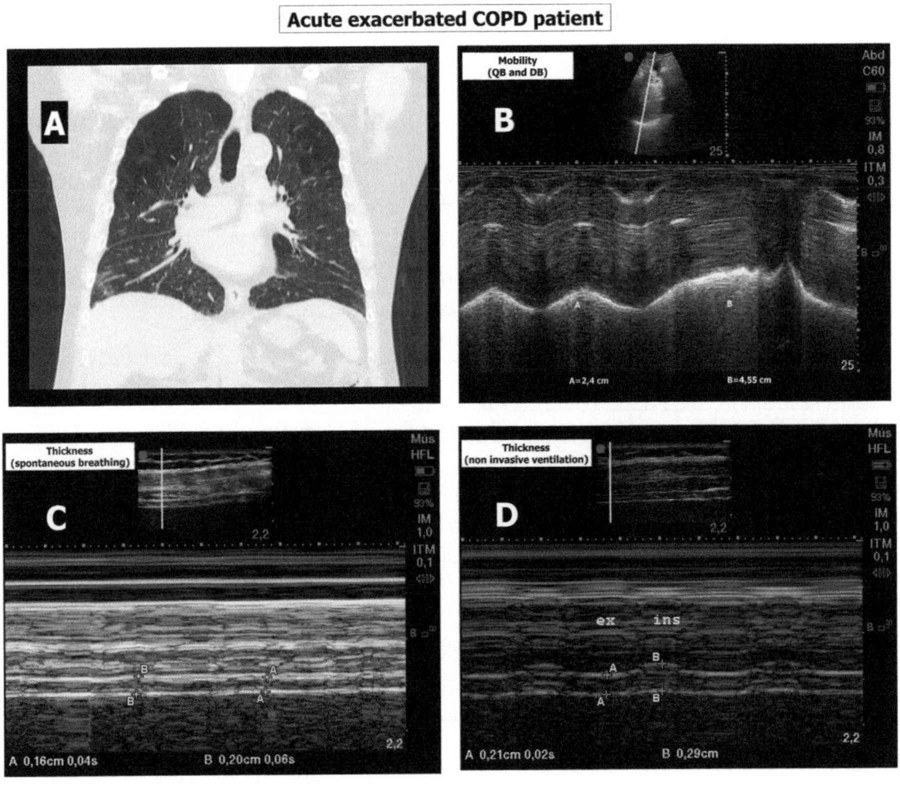

Figure 5.1 Acute exacerbated COPD patient: panel A = Coronal chest CT reconstructions (lung window) demonstrate the classic appearance of visually evident emphysema; panel B = M-mode ultrasonography of the right hemidiaphragm showing mobility during quiet (A) and deep breathing (B); panel C = M-mode ultrasonography of the right hemidiaphragm showing end-expiratory thickness (A) and end-inspiratory thickness (B) during tidal breathing; panel D = M-mode ultrasonography of the right hemidiaphragm showing end-expiratory thickness (A) and end-inspiratory thickness (B) during non-invasive ventilation assisted tidal breathing

45

Table 5.1 Diaphragmatic ultrasound in COPD – main findings and possible clinical relevance

COPD	DUS findings	Clinical relevance
Air trapping		
Dos Santos Yamaguti (10)	• decreased diaphragmatic mobility	• decreased diaphragmatic mobility associated with exercise intolerance and exertional dyspnea • decreased diaphragmatic mobility can be ameliorated by pulmonary rehabilitation improving clinical outcomes
Hyperinflation		
Shiraishi et al. (13)	• decreased diaphragmatic mobility	• decreased diaphragmatic mobility associated with decreased exercise capacity and increased dyspnea due to dynamic lung hyperinflation
Smargiassi (15)	• decreased diaphragmatic thickening	• DUS could be useful to assess lung hyperinflation and the loss of free fat mass in COPD
Chronic overload		
Rittayamai et al. (17)	• increased tidal thickening fraction of the diaphragm during resting breathing)	• decreased diaphragm force reserve ratio
Muscle dysfunction-related factors		
Smargiassi et al. (15)	• decreased diaphragmatic thickening DUS could be useful to assess lung hyperinflation and the loss of free fat mass in COPD	• DUS could be useful to assess the loss of free fat mass in COPD
COPD severity		
Rittayamai et al. (17)	• reduced maximal thickening fraction of the diaphragm and decreased diaphragm force reserve ratio	• poorer diaphragm function was associated with COPD severity, inspiratory capacity (dynamic hyperinflation) and the BODE index • decreased diaphragm force reserve ratio associated with greater chance of exacerbation

(Continued)

Table 5.1 (Continued) Diaphragmatic ultrasound in COPD – main findings and possible clinical relevance

COPD	DUS findings	Clinical relevance
Diaphragmatic function during acute exacerbation of COPD		
Excursion		
Cammarota et al. (24)	• diaphragmatic excursion was greater in NIV successes than in NIV failures	• diaphragmatic excursion could predict NIV failure during acute exacerbation of COPD
Thickness		
Antenora et al. (20) Marchinoi et al. (21)	• diaphragmatic dysfunction (DD) is highly prevalent during acute exacerbation • DD was associated with steroid use and poorer outcomes	• diaphragmatic dysfunction associated with poorer outcomes (NIV failure, longer ICU stay, prolonged MV, need for tracheostomy, and higher ICU mortality

Interstitial Lung Diseases (ILD)

Rationale for Diaphragmatic Dysfunction in ILD

Interstitial lung diseases (ILDs) are a heterogeneous group of inflammatory disorders characterized by fibrosis and inflammation of the lung parenchyma that induces progressive lung volume reduction and stiffness, and pulmonary gas exchange limitations (25), leading to exertional dyspnea and exercise intolerance (26).

Lung stiffness deranges respiratory mechanics in ILD. Respiratory pressure–volume relationship is contracted, even at rest, with reduced inspiratory capacity and IRV. Exercise induces early a critical dynamic constraint because end-inspiratory lung volume encroaches close to the reduced TLC (upper non-linear respiratory pressure–volume relationship), blunting VT expansion. The lung stiffness and the blunted VT expansion elicit high loads over inspiratory muscles to attain ventilation, increasing the inspiratory neural drive to the diaphragm (NMD). To minimize the inspiratory effort (high inspiratory pressures required with poorly compliant lung tissue), ILD patients markedly increase their breathing frequency, typically exhibiting a rapid, shallow breathing pattern during exercise (27).

Often, ILD patients exhibit a preserved inspiratory muscle function reflecting the advantageous inspiratory force generation (lower operating lung volumes decrease the diaphragmatic curvature improving muscle length–tension relationship) and a training effect (chronic increased mechanical load). However, both diaphragmatic weakness (28) and fatigue (29) were demonstrated in ILD, probably related to the myriad of potential adverse factors to muscle function (inflammatory status, hypoxemia, corticosteroid use, physical inactivity, and muscle deconditioning, cachexia, excessive chronic overload) in ILD (26, 27).

DUS in ILD – Diaphragmatic Mobility and Thickness

The respiratory muscles were poorly explored in ILD (30), and few studies employed DUS. He et al. (31) studied the diaphragmatic motion of combined pulmonary fibrosis and emphysema patients ($n = 25$), idiopathic pulmonary fibrosis (IPF; $n = 18$), and COPD ($n = 60$) in comparison with healthy controls ($n = 21$). Diaphragmatic mobility was similar between IPF patients and healthy controls.

However, recently, diaphragmatic dysfunction has been observed in ILD (32–35).

Santana et al. (32) investigated the applicability of DUS in ILD, and compared DUS findings (diaphragmatic mobility and thickness) in ILD patients ($n = 40$) and healthy controls ($n = 16$) and the correlations between diaphragmatic function and lung volumes in ILD. They found that when compared with controls, deep breathing diaphragmatic mobility and the thickening fraction were lower in ILD patients, but diaphragm thickness at FRC (Tdi) was greater in ILD. Diaphragmatic mobility correlated with ILD severity, and FVC values lower than 60% accurately identified diaphragmatic dysfunction on DUS.

Boccatonda et al. (33) investigated the differences between diaphragmatic mobility in IPF patients ($n = 12$) and healthy controls ($n = 12$), and whether there were correlations between diaphragmatic mobility, anthropometric parameters, and respiratory function. They similarly found that deep breathing diaphragmatic mobility was lower in IPF patients than in healthy controls, which was positively correlated with FVC.

The clinical relevance of diaphragmatic dysfunction in ILD was recently explored (34, 35).

Santana et al. (34) compared diaphragmatic function (mobility and thickness) between fibrotic ILD patients (f-ILD; $n = 30$) and healthy controls ($n = 30$), and correlated these findings with dyspnea, exercise tolerance, HRQoL, and lung function. Again, f-ILD cases showed decreased deep breathing diaphragmatic mobility. Compared with healthy controls, f-ILD patients presented greater diaphragm thickness at FRC (Tdi), but lower thickening fraction. Further, deep breathing diaphragmatic mobility and thickness correlated with lung function, exercise tolerance, and HRQoL, but inversely correlated with dyspnea. Most f-ILD cases (70%) presented reduced TF, and these patients had higher dyspnea and exercise desaturation, lower HRQoL and lung function.

Another aspect recently explored in f-ILD patients was whether respiratory muscle incoordination and thoracoabdominal asynchrony (TAA) occur in f-ILD (fibrotic ILD) during exercise and its relationship to lung function and exercise performance (35). The authors showed that during exercise, when compared to controls, f-ILD patients showed increased and early recruitment of the inspiratory scalene muscle and TAA. Compared to f-ILD patients without TAA, f-ILD patients with TAA had less deep breathing diaphragmatic mobility and a trend towards lower thickening fraction, suggesting that the diaphragm dysfunction (reduced mobility and thickening) may represent a dysfunctional diaphragmatic action during exercise, promoting the respiratory muscles incoordination.

Figure 5.2 illustrates the findings of DUS in a healthy subject and a f-ILD patient.

Table 5.2 illustrates the main findings of DUS in ILD and its possible clinical relevance.

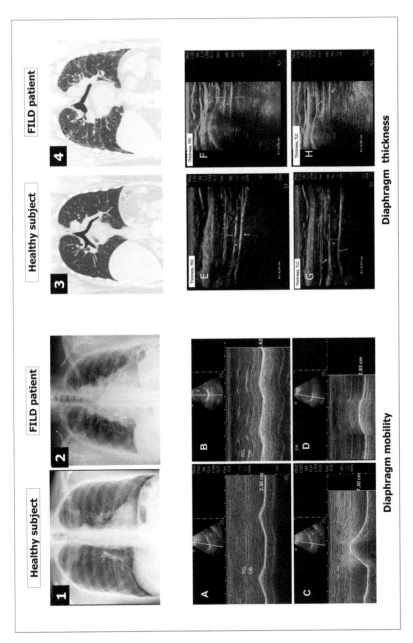

Figure 5.2 Panel of images to compare a healthy subject and a fibrotic ILD patient: The top of the panel shows CXR (Healthy subject in 1 and FILD patient in 2) and images of a chest CT reconstructions (lung window) of a healthy subject (3 – normal appearance) and FILD (4 – classic appearance of lung fibrosis); panels A and C = M-mode ultrasonography of the right hemidiaphragm showing normal mobility during quiet and reduced deep breathing mobility; panels E and G = B-mode ultrasonography of the diaphragm showing normal end-inspiratory thickness (E) and normal maximal thickening (G); panels F and H = B-mode ultrasonography of the diaphragm showing normal end-inspiratory thickness (F) and reduced maximal thickening (H) in a FILD patient

Table 5.2 Diaphragmatic ultrasound in ILD – main findings and possible clinical relevance

ILD	DUS findings	Clinical relevance
Restrictive disorder		
Santana et al. (32) Boccatonda (33)	• reduced deep breathing diaphragmatic mobility	• diaphragmatic mobility correlated with ILD severity *lung function)
Chronic overload		
Santana et al. (32, 34)	• increased diaphragmatic thickness	• "pseudohypertrophy"
Muscle dysfunction		
Santana (34, 35)	• decreased deep breathing diaphragmatic mobility and reduced thickening fraction	• correlated with lung function, exercise tolerance and HRQoL, but inversely correlated with dyspnea • reduced thickening highly prevalent in ILD • may be associated with thoracoabdominal incoordination

Asthma Cystic Fibrosis and Non-cystic Fibrosis Bronchiectasis

Asthma

Respiratory muscle function, diaphragm in particular, was evaluated in a late study by DeBruin et al. (36) who compared the respiratory and limb muscles strength with the muscles' dimensions, assessed by ultrasound, in chronic asthmatic patients ($n = 9$) and healthy subjects ($n = 9$). They found a modestly impaired inspiratory muscle strength and slightly increased diaphragmatic thickness, with preserved quadriceps strength in asthmatic patients. This slightly increased diaphragmatic thickness may indicate muscle hypertrophy.

Cystic Fibrosis (CF)

Many studies investigated diaphragmatic function in CF (37–39). Pinet et al. (37) measured diaphragm and limb muscle function in CF patients with severe respiratory impairment and malnutrition ($n = 18$), and matched controls ($n = 15$). They found that CF patients had diaphragmatic weakness, but thicker diaphragms and abdominal muscles than controls, indicating hypertrophy due to respiratory muscle training. However, the large variability of diaphragm mass suggests that muscle training response does not occur in all CF patients.

Dufresne et al. (38) investigated whether this variability of diaphragm response could reflect the combined and opposite effects of training and systemic inflammation in CF patients ($n = 38$) compared to matched controls ($n = 20$). They showed that CF patients had thicker diaphragms and higher inspiratory muscle strength than controls, consistent with a training effect. Yet, FFM and airway resistance, but not systemic inflammation, were independent predictors of diaphragm thickness, suggesting that the diaphragmatic training occurred in CF despite the presence of inflammation.

However, many adverse factors to the respiratory muscles function (malnutrition, inflammatory status, physical deconditioning, and corticosteroids) are present in chronic respiratory diseases.

Enright et al. (39) assessed the influence of CF severity and FFM on inspiratory muscle function and diaphragm thickness in CF patients ($n = 40$) and matched healthy controls ($n = 30$). They found that CF patients with severe pulmonary disease and low FFM have poor inspiratory muscle function and reduced diaphragm thickness when compared to CF patients with a normal FFM, indicating the adverse influence of reduced physical activity on relaxed and contracted diaphragm thickness and thickening ratio in CF.

Sklar et al. (40) measured the thickening fraction of the diaphragm (TFdi) in exacerbated CF patients ($n = 15$) to compare the effects of high-flow nasal oxygen therapy (HFNT) versus

Table 5.3 Diaphragmatic ultrasound in respiratory diseases – main findings and possible clinical relevance

	DUS findings	Possible clinical relevance
Asthma		
• Overload • De Bruin et al. (36)	• increased thickness ("pseudohypertrophy"?)	• modestly impaired inspiratory muscle strength
Cystic fibrosis		
• Chronic overload/ training • Pinet et al. (37) • Dufresne et al. (38)	• increased thickness (hypertrophy)	• contrasts the systemic adverse effects retaining diaphragmatic function
• Pulmonary disease severity • Enright et al. (39) • Malnutrition (low FFM) • Enright et al. (39)	• reduced diaphragm thickness	• reduction in physical activity, poor inspiratory muscle work capacity and function capabilities
Non-cystic Fibrosis Bronchiectasis		
• Systemic inflammation / infections • Tanriverdi el al (42)	• diaphragm thickness and mobility correlate with disease severity, lung function and physical activity	• DUS may reflect lung function and physical activity

non-invasive ventilation (NIV) in terms of work of breathing. They found that diaphragmatic activity per breath, as assessed by TFdi, was similar between HFNT and NIV. However, according to Corcione et al. (41), TFdi could be only a partial expression of the Work of Breathing (WOB) in CF adults, suggesting that further studies must be performed.

Non-cystic Fibrosis Bronchiectasis

In a recent study, Tanriverdi et al. (42) studied non-cystic fibrosis (non-CF) bronchiectasis patients (n = 38) to assess diaphragm thickness (DT) and mobility (DM) and to investigate their relationship to clinical parameters. DT was related to disease severity, pulmonary function, and physical activity, while DM was related to disease severity and pulmonary function.

Table 5.3 displays the main findings of DUS in asthma, cystic fibrosis, and non-cystic fibrosis bronchiectasis.

Diaphragm Paralysis and DUS Findings

Diaphragm paralysis (DP) is characterized by loss of force generation secondary to the involvement of at least one of the structures: brain central command, phrenic nerves, neuromuscular transmission, and the hemidiaphragms. As a result, the muscle tends to become thin and flaccid, except in diseases of muscle deposits (like amyloidosis). In bilateral diaphragmatic paralysis, the inspiration is attained by the inspiratory intercostal and accessory muscles action pulling and expanding the rib cage, lowering the pleural pressure. During inspiration, the paralyzed diaphragm moves cranially and does not thicken (43).

Considering these functional aspects, the DUS has great relevance for the diagnosis of diaphragm paralysis with high accuracy. Figure 5.3 illustrates the findings of DUS in acute diaphragm paralysis.

Gottesman et al. (44) used DUS to assess DP and showed a reduction of Tdi-exp (< 20mm) and TF (< 20%) in paralyzed hemidiaphragm. The authors reinforce the relevance of performing DUS during deep inspiration, in which some DP patients present even negative values of TF in contrast to the increased values in preserved hemidiaphragm (44). Negative TF was attributed to passive stretching of the paralyzed diaphragm, as also observed in a case report (45) of acute diaphragmatic paralysis, in which TF was negative but Tdi was unaltered, because atrophy may not yet have occurred (45).

This property of inspiratory thickening is important because it is possible to discriminate a recent involvement of diaphragm (preserved Tdi but reduced TF) from chronic dysfunction (Tdi and TF reduced). Callefi-Pereira (46) confirmed the diminished thickness (Tdi, Tdi-insp, and TF) in patients with chronic unilateral diaphragm, and pointed out the force generation was impaired even in the preserved hemidiaphragm.

Diaphragm mobility during normal or deep breathing is a very sensitive finding in DP. Different studies have already shown a consistent reduction of mobility in both situations, when contrasted to the preserved hemidiaphragm or healthy controls (46–48). DUS shows a specific pattern with a paradoxical mobility during voluntary sniffing (M-mode) in DP. Interestingly, this paradoxical mobility also occurs in stress condition,

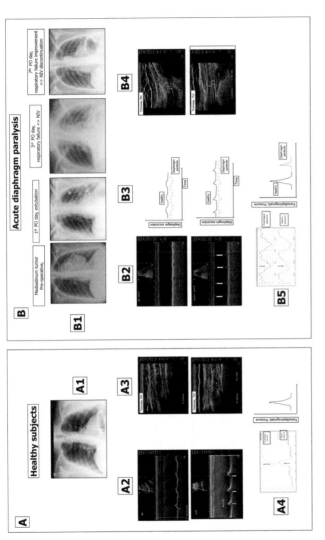

Figure 5.3 Panel of images to compare a healthy subject (A) and a patient with post-operative acute diaphragm paralysis (B). Panel A1 shows CXR (healthy subject). Panel A2 displays M-mode ultrasonography of the right hemidiaphragm showing normal mobility during quiet and sniff manoeuvre. Panel A3 displays B-mode ultrasonography of the diaphragm showing normal end-inspiratory thickness (FRC) and normal thickening (TF) and maximal thickness (TLC). Panel A4 displays the respiratory pressures (esophageal and gastric pressures, at left) during a sniff manoeuvre and an illustrative graph of normal transdiaphragmatic pressure (right); Panel B1 shows the sequence of CXR (as designated in each one, from pre-operative status, and subsequently, until the suspicion of diaphragm paralysis at third PO, and recovery at seventh PO). Panel B2 displays M-mode ultrasonography of the left hemidiaphragm showing paradoxal mobility during quiet and sniff manoeuvre. Panel A3 displays an illustrative graphic of expected normal diaphragm mobility (black dashed line) and abnormal (paralyzed) diaphragm mobility (red dashed line). Panel B4 displays B-mode ultrasonography of the left paralyzed diaphragm showing normal end-inspiratory thickness (FRC, indicative of no atrophy), but decreased thickening (diminished TF) and reduced maximal thickness (TLC). Panel B5 displays the respiratory pressures (denoting negative inspiratory gastric pressures – paradoxal, at left) during a sniff manoeuvre and an illustrative graphic of expected normal transdiaphragmatic pressure (black dashed line) and abnormal (paralyzed) transdiaphragmatic pressure (red dashed line)

53

like exercise as demonstrated by Callefi-Pereira (49), who found a negative gastric pressure (in accordance with paradoxical mobility) during exercise progression, in contrast to sustained positivation in healthy individuals. Finally, these DP patients presented reduced transdiaphragmatic pressure, higher inspiratory muscle recruitment, and higher dyspnea during exercise (49).

DUS is a valuable tool to monitor the recovery of diaphragm paralysis. Summerhill et al. (50) evaluated patients with DP ($n = 16$) up to 60 months, using diaphragmatic TF and found that 43% recovered their diaphragmatic function (mean recovery time of 14.9 ± 6.1 months), whereas the remaining patients did not.

Even in the acute follow-up, Ultrasonography may be useful. In surgeries which involve neck dissection, DUS was able to identify atrophy in patients at one month post procedure (51).

DP may also complicate the postoperative cardiac or thoracic surgery. Lerolle et al. (52) studied patients requiring prolonged MV (> 7 days) after cardiac surgery ($n = 28$) compared to a control group ($n = 20$; patients with an uncomplicated postoperative course). They measured the transdiaphragmatic pressure (Pdi), the Gilbert index (ratio between gastric pressure during inspiration, to the amplitude of Pdi during inspiration), which evaluates the diaphragm's contribution to respiratory pressures (normal values > 0.30; values ≤ 0 indicate severe diaphragmatic dysfunction). Diaphragmatic mobility during maximal inspiratory effort (Demax) was measured with DUS. Among the 28 patients receiving prolonged MV, 27 patients had a reduced Pdi, and eight patients had Gilbert indexes ≤ 0 (severe DD) in which DEmax was lower than in patients with a Gilbert index > 0. Additionally, during maximal inspiratory effort, a diaphragmatic mobility < 25 mm accurately predicted a Gilbert index $\leq$ 0 (AUC of 0.93). The DEmax was > 25 mm in all the patients with an uncomplicated course.

Table 5.4 shows the main findings of DUS in diaphragm paralysis.

Figure 5.4 illustrates the findings of DUS in a healthy subject and a patient with a chronic diaphragm paralysis.

Table 5.4 Diaphragmatic ultrasound in diaphragm paralysis

Time course	Excursion	Thickness and thickening
Acute or subacute paralysis	• diaphragmatic excursion reduced or absent or paradoxal DE (45)	• unaltered Tdi (Tdi > 0.15 cm) with abnormal TF (TF < 20% even negative) (45) • Tdi may be unaltered (45)
Chronic paralysis	• diaphragmatic excursion reduced, or absent, or paradoxal during QB (47, 48) • diaphragmatic excursion reduced, absent, or paradoxal during DB and Sniff (47)	• atrophy: Tdi < 0.11 – 0.12 cm (LLN) (46) • atrophy and reduced TF (< 20%) (44) • TF < 20%, even negative (44)
Diaphragm paralysis recovery		
	• DUS may follow the recovery of diaphragm paralysis (50)	

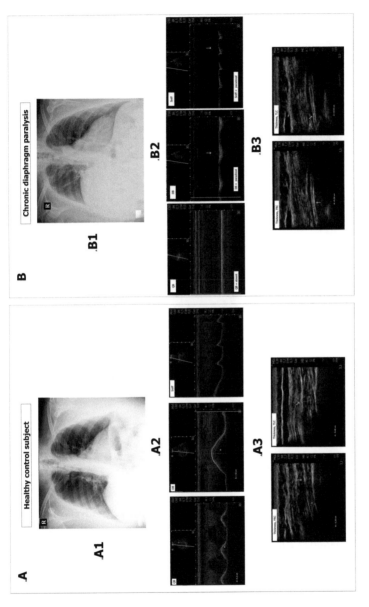

Figure 5.4 Panel of images to compare a healthy subject (A) and a patient with chronic diaphragm paralysis (B). Panel A1 shows CXR (healthy subject). Panel A2 displays M-mode ultrasonography of the right hemidiaphragm showing normal mobility during quiet and deep breathing, and sniff manoeuvre. Panel A3 displays B-mode ultrasonography of the diaphragm showing normal end-inspiratory thickness (FRC), normal thickening (TF) and maximal thickness (TLC). Panel B1 shows the CXR of a chronic paralyzed diaphragm. Panel B2 displays M-mode ultrasonography of the right paralyzed hemidiaphragm showing absent mobility during quiet breathing and paradoxal mobility during deep breathing and sniff manoeuvre. Panel B3 displays B-mode ultrasonography of the right paralyzed diaphragm showing reduced end-inspiratory thickness (FRC, indicative of atrophy) and decreased thickening (reduced TF and maximal thickness – TLC)

Key points

Diaphragm Ultrasound
o provides a real-time, non-invasive method for assessing the diaphragm.
o may disclose several aspects of diaphragmatic function and structure.

In COPD
o diaphragmatic function assessed by ultrasound may be useful to monitor air trapping, hyperinflation, and loss of free fat mass.
o diaphragmatic function assessed by ultrasound may be associated with exercise tolerance and exertional dyspnea.
o diaphragmatic function assessed by DUS was able to accurately identify COPD patients who improved after PR.
o diaphragmatic function assessed by ultrasound may predict clinical outcomes during acute exacerbations and disclose diaphragmatic dysfunction

In ILD
o diaphragmatic function assessed by ultrasound may be useful to monitor lung function.
o diaphragmatic function assessed by ultrasound may disclose diaphragmatic dysfunction.
o diaphragmatic function assessed by ultrasound may be associated with exercise tolerance, exertional dyspnea, and health-related quality of life.

In Cystic Fibrosis
o diaphragmatic function assessed by ultrasound may be useful to monitor chronic overload/training effect (hypertrophy).
o diaphragmatic function assessed by ultrasound may be useful to monitor the contrast of the training effect in opposite to the systemic adverse effects (malnutrition, systemic inflammation, disease severity).

In Diaphragm Paralysis
o diaphragmatic function assessed by ultrasound may be useful to establish the diagnosis.
o diaphragmatic function assessed by ultrasound may be useful to monitor the recovery.

References

1. O'Donnell DE, Elbehairy AF, Berton DC, Domnik NJ, Neder JA. Advances in the evaluation of respiratory pathophysiology during exercise in chronic lung diseases. *Frontiers in Physiology.* 2017;8:82.

2. Faisal A, Alghamdi BJ, Ciavaglia CE, Elbehairy AF, Webb KA, Ora J, et al. Common mechanisms of dyspnea in chronic interstitial and obstructive lung disorders. *American Journal of Respiratory and Critical Care Medicine.* 2016;193(3):299–309.

3. Cardenas LZ, Santana PV, Caruso P, de Carvalho CRR, de Albuquerque ALP. Diaphragmatic ultrasound correlates with inspiratory muscle strength and pulmonary function in healthy subjects. *Ultrasound in Medicine & Biology.* 2018;44(4):786–93.

4. O'Donnell DE. Hyperinflation, dyspnea, and exercise intolerance in chronic obstructive pulmonary disease. *Proceedings of the American Thoracic Society.* 2006;3(2):180–4.

5. De Troyer A. Effect of hyperinflation on the diaphragm. *European Respiratory Journal.* 1997;10(3):708–13.

6. Kim HC, Mofarrahi M, Hussain SN. Skeletal muscle dysfunction in patients with chronic obstructive pulmonary disease. *International Journal of Chronic Obstructive Pulmonary Disease.* 2008;3(4):637.

7. Barreiro E, De La Puente B, Minguella J, Corominas JM, Serrano S, Hussain SN, et al. Oxidative stress and respiratory muscle dysfunction in severe chronic obstructive pulmonary disease. *American Journal of Respiratory and Critical Care Medicine.* 2005;171(10):1116–24.

8. Levine S, Nguyen T, Kaiser LR, Rubinstein NA, Maislin G, Gregory C, et al. Human diaphragm remodeling associated with chronic obstructive pulmonary disease: clinical implications. *American Journal of Respiratory and Critical Care Medicine.* 2003;168(6):706–13.

9. Ottenheijm CA, Heunks LM, Sieck GC, Zhan W-Z, Jansen SM, Degens H, et al. Diaphragm dysfunction in chronic obstructive pulmonary disease. *American Journal of Respiratory and Critical Care Medicine.* 2005;172(2):200–5.

10. Dos Santos Yamaguti WP, Paulin E, Shibao S, Chammas MC, Salge JM, Ribeiro M, et al. Air trapping: the major factor limiting diaphragm mobility in chronic obstructive pulmonary disease patients. *Respirology.* 2008;13(1):138–44.

11. Scheibe N, Sosnowski N, Pinkhasik A, Vonderbank S, Bastian A. Sonographic evaluation of diaphragmatic dysfunction in COPD patients. *International Journal of Chronic Obstructive Pulmonary Disease.* 2015;10:1925.

12. Paulin E, Yamaguti W, Chammas M, Shibao S, Stelmach R, Cukier A, et al. Influence of diaphragmatic mobility on exercise tolerance and dyspnea in patients with COPD. *Respiratory Medicine.* 2007;101(10):2113–8.

13. Shiraishi M, Higashimoto Y, Sugiya R, Mizusawa H, Takeda Y, Fujita S, et al. Diaphragmatic excursion correlates with exercise capacity and dynamic hyperinflation in COPD patients. *ERJ Open Research.* 2020;6(4).

14. Baria MR, Shahgholi L, Sorenson EJ, Harper CJ, Lim KG, Strommen JA, et al. B-mode ultrasound assessment of diaphragm structure and function in patients with COPD. *Chest.* 2014;146(3):680–5.

15. Smargiassi A, Inchingolo R, Tagliaboschi L, Berardino ADM, Valente S, Corbo GM. Ultrasonographic assessment of the diaphragm in chronic obstructive pulmonary disease patients: relationships with pulmonary function and the influence of body composition-a pilot study. *Respiration.* 2014;87(5):364–71.

16. Okura K, Iwakura M, Shibata K, Kawagoshi A, Sugawara K, Takahashi H, et al. Diaphragm thickening assessed by ultrasonography is lower than healthy adults in patients with chronic obstructive pulmonary disease. *The Clinical Respiratory Journal.* 2020;14(6):521–6.

17. Rittayamai N, Chuaychoo B, Tscheikuna J, Dres M, Goligher EC, Brochard L. Ultrasound evaluation of diaphragm force reserve in patients with chronic obstructive pulmonary disease. *Annals of the American Thoracic Society.* 2020;17(10):1222–30.

18. Corbellini C, Boussuges A, Villafañe JH, Zocchi L. Diaphragmatic mobility loss in subjects with moderate to very severe COPD may improve after in-patient pulmonary rehabilitation. *Respiratory Care.* 2018;63(10):1271–80.

19. Crimi C, Heffler E, Augelletti T, Campisi R, Noto A, Vancheri C, et al. Utility of ultrasound assessment of diaphragmatic function before and after pulmonary rehabilitation in COPD patients. *International Journal of Chronic Obstructive Pulmonary Disease.* 2018;13:3131.

20. Antenora F, Fantini R, Iattoni A, Castaniere I, Sdanganelli A, Livrieri F, et al. Prevalence and outcomes of diaphragmatic dysfunction assessed by ultrasound technology during acute exacerbation of COPD: a pilot study. *Respirology.* 2017;22(2):338–44.

21. Marchioni A, Castaniere I, Tonelli R, Fantini R, Fontana M, Tabbì L, et al. Ultrasound-assessed diaphragmatic impairment is a predictor of outcomes in patients with acute exacerbation of chronic obstructive pulmonary disease undergoing noninvasive ventilation. *Critical Care.* 2018;22(1):1–9.

22. Abbas A, Embarak S, Walaa M, Lutfy SM. Role of diaphragmatic rapid shallow breathing index in predicting weaning outcome in patients with acute exacerbation of COPD. *International Journal of Chronic Obstructive Pulmonary Disease.* 2018;13:1655.

23. Lim SY, Lim G, Lee YJ, Cho YJ, Park JS, Yoon HI, et al. Ultrasound assessment of diaphragmatic function during acute exacerbation of chronic obstructive pulmonary disease: a pilot study. *International Journal of Chronic Obstructive Pulmonary Disease.* 2019;14:2479.

24. Cammarota G, Sguazzotti I, Zanoni M, Messina A, Colombo D, Vignazia GL, et al. Diaphragmatic ultrasound assessment in subjects with acute hypercapnic respiratory failure admitted to the emergency department. *Respiratory Care.* 2019;64(12):1469–77.

25. Chetta A, Marangio E, Olivieri D. Pulmonary function testing in interstitial lung diseases. *Respiration.* 2004;71(3):209–13.

26. Holland AE. Exercise limitation in interstitial lung disease-mechanisms, significance and therapeutic options. *Chronic Respiratory Disease.* 2010;7(2):101–11.

27. Panagiotou M, Polychronopoulos V, Strange C. Respiratory and lower limb muscle function in interstitial lung disease. *Chronic Respiratory Disease.* 2016;13(2):162–72.

28. Walterspacher S, Schlager D, Walker DJ, Müller-Quernheim J, Windisch W, Kabitz H-J. Respiratory muscle function in interstitial lung disease. European Respiratory Journal. 2013;42(1):211–9.

29. Elia D, Kelly JL, Martolini D, Renzoni EA, Boutou AK, Chetta A, et al. Respiratory muscle fatigue following exercise in patients with interstitial lung disease. *Respiration.* 2013;85(3):220–7.

30. Baldi BG, Salge JM. Respiratory muscles in interstitial lung disease: poorly explored and poorly understood. *Jornal Brasileiro de Pneumologia.* 2016;42(2):82–3.

31. He L, Zhang W, Zhang J, Cao L, Gong L, Ma J, et al. Diaphragmatic motion studied by M-mode ultrasonography in combined pulmonary fibrosis and emphysema. *Lung.* 2014;192(4):553–61.

32. Santana PV, Prina E, Albuquerque ALP, Carvalho CRR, Caruso P. Identifying decreased diaphragmatic mobility and diaphragm thickening in interstitial lung disease: the utility of ultrasound imaging. *Jornal Brasileiro de Pneumologia*. 2016;42(2):88–94.

33. Boccatonda A, Decorato V, Cocco G, Marinari S, Schiavone C. Ultrasound evaluation of diaphragmatic mobility in patients with idiopathic lung fibrosis: a pilot study. *Multidisciplinary Respiratory Medicine*. 2019;14(1):1–6.

34. Santana PV, Cardenas LZ, de Albuquerque ALP, de Carvalho CRR, Caruso P. Diaphragmatic ultrasound findings correlate with dyspnea, exercise tolerance, health-related quality of life and lung function in patients with fibrotic interstitial lung disease. *BMC Pulmonary Medicine*. 2019;19(1):1–10.

35. Santana PV, Cardenas LZ, Ferreira JG, de Carvalho CRR, de Albuquerque ALP, Caruso P. Thoracoabdominal asynchrony associates with exercise intolerance in fibrotic interstitial lung diseases. *Respirology*. 2021;26:673–682.

36. De Bruin P, Ueki J, Watson A, Pride N. Size and strength of the respiratory and quadriceps muscles in patients with chronic asthma. *European Respiratory Journal*. 1997;10(1):59–64.

37. Pinet C, Cassart M, Scillia P, Lamotte M, Knoop C, Casimir G, et al. Function and bulk of respiratory and limb muscles in patients with cystic fibrosis. *American Journal of Respiratory and Critical Care Medicine*. 2003;168(8):989–94.

38. Dufresne V, Knoop C, Van Muylem A, Malfroot A, Lamotte M, Opdekamp C, et al. Effect of systemic inflammation on inspiratory and limb muscle strength and bulk in cystic fibrosis. *American Journal of Respiratory and Critical Care Medicine*. 2009;180(2):153–8.

39. Enright S, Chatham K, Ionescu AA, Unnithan VB, Shale DJ. The influence of body composition on respiratory muscle, lung function and diaphragm thickness in adults with cystic fibrosis. *Journal of Cystic Fibrosis*. 2007;6(6):384–90.

40. Sklar MC, Dres M, Rittayamai N, West B, Grieco DL, Telias I, et al. High-flow nasal oxygen versus noninvasive ventilation in adult patients with cystic fibrosis: a randomized crossover physiological study. *Annals of Intensive Care*. 2018;8(1):1–9.

41. Corcione N, Buonpensiero P, Esquinas AM. High flow oxygen therapy and the work of breathing assessed by thickening fraction of the diaphragm (TFdi): just a side of the moon in cystic fibrosis patients? *Annals of Translational Medicine*. 2019;7(3):58.

42. Tanriverdi A, Savci S, Mese M, Gezer NS, Kahraman BO, Sevinc C. Diaphragmatic ultrasound in non-cystic fibrosis bronchiectasis: relationship to clinical parameters. *Ultrasound in Medicine & Biology*. 2021;47(4):902–9.

43. Gibson G. Diaphragmatic paresis: pathophysiology, clinical features, and investigation. *Thorax*. 1989;44(11):960.

44. Gottesman E, McCool FD. Ultrasound evaluation of the paralyzed diaphragm. *American Journal of Respiratory and Critical Care Medicine*. 1997;155(5):1570–4.

45. Santana PV, Prina E, Caruso P, Carvalho CR, Albuquerque AL. Dyspnea of unknown cause. Think about diaphragm. *Annals of the American Thoracic Society*. 2014;11(10):1656–9.

46. Caleffi-Pereira M, Pletsch-Assunção R, Cardenas LZ, Santana PV, Ferreira JG, Iamonti VC, et al. Unilateral diaphragm paralysis: a dysfunction restricted not just to one hemidiaphragm. *BMC Pulmonary Medicine*. 2018;18(1):1–9.

47. Boussuges A, Brégeon F, Blanc P, Gil JM, Poirette L. Characteristics of the paralysed diaphragm studied by M-mode ultrasonography. *Clinical Physiology and Functional Imaging*. 2019;39(2):143–9.

48. Lloyd T, Tang Y, Benson M, King S. Diaphragmatic paralysis: the use of M mode ultrasound for diagnosis in adults. *Spinal Cord*. 2006;44(8):505–8.

49. Pereira MC, Cardenas LZ, Ferreira JG, Iamonti VC, Santana PV, Apanavicius A, et al. Unilateral diaphragmatic paralysis: inspiratory muscles, breathlessness and exercise capacity. *ERJ Open Research*. 2021;7(1):00357-2019.

50. Summerhill EM, El-Sameed YA, Glidden TJ, McCool FD. Monitoring recovery from diaphragm paralysis with ultrasound. *Chest*. 2008;133(3):737–43.

51. Santana AFSG, Caruso P, Santana PV, Porto GCLM, Kowalski LP, Vartanian JG. Inspiratory muscle weakness, diaphragm immobility and diaphragm atrophy after neck dissection. *European Archives of Oto-Rhino-Laryngology*. 2018;275(5):1227–34.

52. Lerolle N, Guérot E, Dimassi S, Zegdi R, Faisy C, Fagon J-Y, et al. Ultrasonographic diagnostic criterion for severe diaphragmatic dysfunction after cardiac surgery. *Chest*. 2009;135(2):401–7.

Assessment of Diaphragm Dysfunction in Mechanically Ventilated Patients

Quentin Fossé and Martin Dres

Introduction

The diaphragm is a respiratory muscle of importance. Along with the extra-diaphragm respiratory muscles, it enables the ventilation function of the chest wall and the mobilization of the air into the alveoli. In mechanically ventilated patients, the respiratory muscles are frequently unloaded which is likely to lead – among other risk factors – to a time-dependent dysfunction. The diaphragm function is usually defined as its capacity to generate pressure, namely the transdiaphragmatic pressure. A growing body of evidence brought into light that diaphragm dysfunction is highly prevalent in mechanically ventilated patients and that it is associated with a poor prognosis, in particular at the time of liberation from mechanical ventilation. Diaphragm dysfunction is responsible for a prolonged duration of mechanical ventilation, prolonged weaning and increased length of stay, and negatively influences

DOI: 10.1201/9781003128694-9

morbidity and intensive care unit (ICU) and hospital mortality.[1, 2] Therefore, monitoring the diaphragm function appears as a major clinical question. It may facilitate the detection of the disease and the implementation of protective measures.[3] This chapter aims to provide a detailed and practical review of the assessment techniques of the diaphragm function in mechanically ventilated patients.

Diaphragm Dysfunction

An Underestimated Disease in the ICU

Assessing the diaphragm function in the ICU is challenging. It may explain the scarcity of available data looking at the prevalence of diaphragm dysfunction which has been underestimated for a long time.[1, 4–6] It affects more than 60% of patients at the early phase[1] and up to 80% of those exposed to prolonged mechanical ventilation.[7–9] This high prevalence was reported by Demoule et al. within the first 24 hours after initiation of mechanical ventilation[1] and by Dres et al. in patients ready to undergo a spontaneous breathing trial.[9] These last two studies used the reference technique (magnetic stimulation of the phrenic nerves) to assess the diaphragm function. When diaphragm dysfunction is identified by using ultrasound criteria the prevalence seems lower – between 25 and 35%[4, 10] – but the definition is less arbitrary than with the reference technique and varies according to studies. Nonetheless, this high prevalence justifies suspecting and sometimes confirming the presence of diaphragm dysfunction in case of difficult or prolonged weaning from mechanical ventilation. Accordingly, it also implies the need to develop and implement easy-to-use devices and tools. As detailed further, the reference technique to assess the diaphragm function relies on the phrenic nerves stimulation technique that is not widely available. Therefore, attention has been raised by emerging techniques such as diaphragm ultrasound and diaphragm electrical activity continuous monitoring.

A Disease with Common Risk Factors

Different risk factors for diaphragm dysfunction are encountered before and during the ICU course explaining that on one hand, the diaphragm dysfunction may pre-exist and precipitate the ICU admission and mechanical ventilation's need. On the other hand, the diaphragm function may also worsen during the ICU stay.[1] In the sickest patients, it is likely that multiple risk factors hit simultaneously. Some are present before the ICU admission (sepsis, shock, excessive respiratory loads) while others develop during the ICU stay (use of mechanical ventilation, medications).[4, 11] Animal studies have shown the negative impact of forced rest imposed by controlled mechanical ventilation on the diaphragm function.[12, 13] Accordingly, the term ventilator induced diaphragm dysfunction (VIDD) has been defined as a decrease capacity of the diaphragm to generate a pressure that is solely due to mechanical ventilation.[13] However, patients in the ICU are frequently exposed to confounding risk factors which may justify the use of the term "critical illness associated diaphragm dysfunction" instead of VIDD.[4] As animal studies have shown, it is now established that mechanical ventilation induced respiratory muscle unloading leads to structural and functional time dependent alterations of the diaphragm.[14] Similar findings have been reported in critically ill patients.[7, 11, 15, 16] Conversely, it has been suggested that respiratory distress-induced respiratory muscles overactivity may also induce diaphragm dysfunction.[16-18] This is an interesting hypothesis that has, however, not yet been documented in critically ill patients.

A Disease Associated with Clinical Outcomes

Irrespective of whether it is present at admission[1] or at a later stage,[3, 4, 8, 10] diaphragm dysfunction is a marker of illness severity and of poor prognosis. At the early stage of critical illness, diaphragm dysfunction is analogous to any other form of organ dysfunction and its presence is associated with higher mortality.[1] To what extent diaphragm dysfunction can contribute to a poor prognosis has not been elucidated. Importantly, diaphragm dysfunction can improve despite exposure to mechanical ventilation.[19] Nevertheless, the time of course and the determinants of the recovery need to be clarified in further studies. At the time of liberation from mechanical ventilation, diaphragm function is an important determinant of weaning outcome. In isolation, diaphragm dysfunction is usually not sufficient to precipitate respiratory failure and weaning failure, but in the presence of high ventilatory demands or deteriorating respiratory mechanics it may rapidly result in weaning or extubation failure. In the study by Kim and co-workers who used ultrasound to detect diaphragm dysfunction, diaphragm dysfunction was associated with a longer weaning time (401 hours vs. 90 hours, p < 0.01).[10] However, diaphragm dysfunction can also be present in patients who are successfully liberated from ventilation.[8, 20] Of note, some studies indicate that a substantial proportion of patients (up to 44%) can be successfully weaned from the ventilator despite having diaphragm dysfunction.[1, 7] This is not surprising as many patients with chronic diaphragm dysfunction do not require mechanical ventilation.[21, 22] While diaphragm dysfunction might limit exercise capacity, the clinical consequences of diaphragm dysfunction in successfully liberated patients is uncertain. However, the impact of respiratory muscles dysfunction (not specifically the diaphragm) after critical illness may be of importance since it is associated with worse long-term outcomes.[23, 24] Some findings suggest a high risk of hospital readmission in patients with chronic respiratory failure in case of respiratory muscle dysfunction (not only the diaphragm) seven days after ICU discharge.[23] By contrast, in a non-selected population of ICU patients, Saccheri et al. reported that diaphragm dysfunction is not associated with long-term survival (two years) whereas intensive care unit-acquired weakness had a significant impact.[25]

When Evaluating the Diaphragm Function?

Patients presenting with respiratory distress exhibit important inspiratory efforts. The latter may be responsible for respiratory muscles over-activity which may result in diaphragm injury.[16] Orozco-Levi et al. observed that diaphragm overactivity induced by intense inspiratory efforts can lead to histological signs of diaphragm injury in healthy patients.[18] In addition, higher risk of non-invasive ventilation failure has been documented in patients with diaphragm dysfunction.[26] These studies suggest that monitoring the diaphragm function of patients with respiratory distress may be of interest to evaluate the risk of diaphragm overactivity. Whether it may lead to a clinical decision (intubation) remains to be established.

Diaphragm function may also be monitored under mechanical ventilation. It is now demonstrated that respiratory muscles unloading induced by mechanical ventilation is responsible for a time-dependent alteration of contractile properties of the diaphragm.[12, 14] Tailoring the level of respiratory assistance according to the diaphragm function could mitigate the risk of diaphragm disuse. Conversely, as described above, avoiding intense respiratory efforts could be necessary to prevent the occurrence of diaphragm injury and subsequent dysfunction. Taking into account both the effects of excessive ventilatory assistance on the risk of diaphragm dysfunction and the effects of insufficient ventilatory assistance on the risk of patient self-inflicted lung injury, the main objective of diaphragm function monitoring would be to closely tailor the appropriate level of assistance to the patient's needs and comfort. Thus, the monitoring of the diaphragm function of mechanically ventilated patients addresses the concept of diaphragm-protective ventilation.[27, 28] The latter has not to be opposed to that of lung-protective ventilation. It should be considered as part of its extension.[28] It is important to note that the clinical impact of the diaphragm protective ventilation approach has not been yet investigated. Further studies will have to evaluate the feasibility and efficacy of this strategy.

Last, evaluating the diaphragm function may also be interesting in patients facing weaning failure.[29, 30] Diaphragm dysfunction is associated with weaning failure and an increased duration of mechanical ventilation.[31, 32] Monitoring the diaphragm function at the time of weaning is particularly of interest after cardiac or thoracic surgery which represents an independent risk factor for diaphragm dysfunction. The latter cause phrenic lesions, most often by direct damage to the phrenic nerves at the pericardium.[33, 34]

How Is the Diaphragm Function Defined?

The diaphragm is a thin, dome-shaped musculotendinous membrane stretched between the thorax and the abdominal cavity. Under physiological conditions, the diaphragm acts like a piston in a syringe. The main role of the diaphragm is to shorten and to generate a driving air-flow pressure. However, the latter cannot be easily measured. From a physiological point of view, diaphragm dysfunction can thus be defined by a decrease in its capacity to generate a pressure. This definition is the most used in clinical practice.[35]

Which Methods to Assess the Diaphragm Function?

Different methods have been developed to assess the diaphragm function in the ICU patient.[36] The most physiological method is to measure the transdiaphragmatic pressure but it requires the use of esophageal and gastric balloons. This can be measured under different conditions: during a maximal inspiratory effort, or during a standardized magnetic stimulation of the phrenic nerves which has the main advantage of being independent from the patient's cooperation. It can be measured directly at the mouth (with a nose-clip), at the tip of the endotracheal tube, or by measuring esophageal and gastric pressures. The diaphragm function can also be approached by ultrasound which allows a visual and direct measurement. The measurement of the electrical activity of the muscle, through surface or transesophageal approach, can be used in order to quantify the muscle activity.[37]

Diaphragm Pressure-Generating Capacity

By contracting, shortening, and generating a force, diaphragm contraction generates intrathoracic negative pressure driving inspiratory flow while at the same time the diaphragm lowers and compresses the abdominal cavity content. These pressure changes are specific to the diaphragm. Indeed the diaphragm is the only muscle that can simultaneously increase gastric and decrease intrathoracic pressure (Figures 6.1 and 6.2).

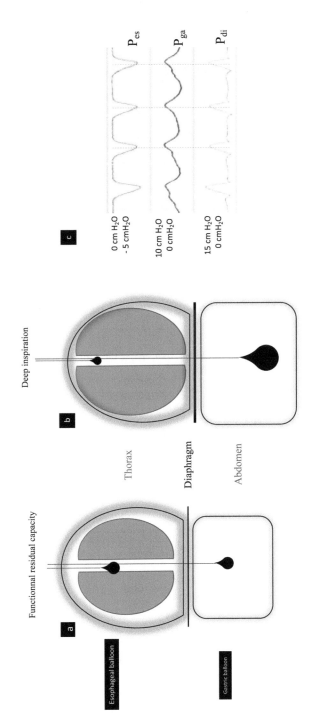

Figure 6.1 During inspiration, the diaphragm contracts, thickens and displaces caudally (panel b) generating simultaneously negative pleural pressure, estimated by the esophageal pressure (panel c, pink tracing) and positive abdominal pressure (panel c, blue tracing) resulting in transdiaphragmatic pressure (panel C, green tracing) computed as Pdi = Pga - Pes

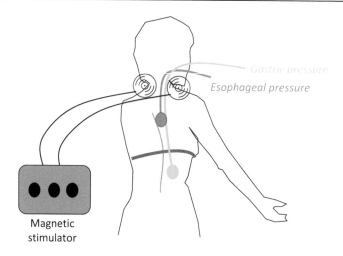

Figure 6.2 Schematic picture of the pressures measured in response to a magnetic anterior phrenic nerves stimulation. Transdiaphragmatic pressure requires the use of gastric and esophageal pressure

Inspiratory Pressure Recorded at the Mouth

Inspiratory pressure recorded at the mouth is a global and integrative approach of the inspiratory system including the diaphragm but also the extra diaphragm respiratory muscles. It is performed by measuring the pressure sustained for one second during a maximum static inspiratory effort (PImax).[35] PI_{max} is a simple measurement but two points should be noted. First, it requires the full collaboration of the patient who must perform a strong inspiratory effort which can be challenging for critically ill patients. Second, it is not specific to the diaphragm function; it represents the pressure provided by all the respiratory muscles. This technique may be adapted to the patients under invasive mechanical ventilation even in case of poor level of consciousness by using a one-way valve allowing expiration but not inspiration.[38–40] It leads the patient to provide increasing inspiratory efforts.[39, 41] Sahn and Lakshminarayan suggested that a PImax cut-off value higher than -30 cmH$_2$O is associated with successful weaning.[42] Patients unable to provide values below -20 cmH$_2$O are more likely to fail weaning.[42]

Transdiaphragmatic Pressure

Transdiaphragmatic pressure is a specific assessment of the diaphragm function. It requires esophageal and gastric balloons inflated with a few millilitres of air and connected to pressure transducers. Thus, simultaneous intra-thoracic and intra-abdominal pressure signals are recorded. The resulting pressure, namely the transdiaphragmatic pressure (Pdi), is defined by the difference between the gastric and esophageal pressures[43] (Figure 6.2). The greater the Pdi, the better the diaphragm function. It is recognized as a physiological and quantitative marker of the diaphragm function.[35] Pdi_{max} defined as Pdi during a maximal effort, seems to be the most physiological approach.[3, 41] In order to standardize the evaluation, endotracheal pressure (Ptr) and Pdi can be measured in response to a bilateral anterior magnetic phrenic nerve stimulation (BAMPS). Instead of measuring Pdi that requires esophageal and gastric balloons, it is acceptable to measure changes in endotracheal pressure in response to magnetic phrenic nerve stimulation (Ptr,stim).[41] Based on previous data[1, 7], a Ptr,stim below -11 cmH$_2$O corresponds to a diaphragm dysfunction. While BAMPS provides a rigorous assessment of the diaphragm function, it is only available in expert centres and requires a costly equipment precluding its generalization.

Ultrasound Assessment

Recent years have been marked by an increasing use of diaphragm ultrasound in the ICU. It is a safe, radiation-free, non-invasive, and widely available technique. Several studies have investigated ultrasound monitoring of the diaphragm function.[44, 45] When the diaphragm contracts, it changes the muscle stiffness, it shorts, thickens and displaces caudally. Ultrasound offers two descriptive approaches of the diaphragm function. The intercostal approach is performed at the apposition zone, a vertical portion of the muscle, in contact with the internal part of the rib grid. This approach provides information on muscle thickness and thickening fraction (TFdi), the latter is computed as the difference between the end-inspiratory thickness and the end-expiratory thickness divided by the end-expiratory thickness. The second, the subcostal approach, evaluates the caudal displacement of the diaphragm dome, the part of the muscle separating the thorax with the abdominal compartment. This caudal movement during inspiration is the excursion (EXdi).[44] EXdi is associated with high intra- and inter-observer reliability and normal values are available for healthy adults and children, and patients.[46, 47] Practical modalities are not developed in this section since EXdi and TFdi have already been discussed in other chapters of this textbook. Importantly, for convenience and echogenicity reasons, diaphragm ultrasound assessment mainly focuses on the right hemidiaphragm and the large majority of published data refer to this side.[3, 46] To avoid underestimation of the diaphragm function, it is preferrable to measure the diaphragm excursion with the lower ventilatory assistance. EXdi can only be interpreted during non-assisted breathing; otherwise the downward displacement of the diaphragm may reflect passive insufflation of the chest by the ventilator.

EXdi measures diaphragm caudal displacement during inspiration. Cut-off values to determine diaphragm dysfunction vary across studies.[8, 33, 48, 49] In healthy subjects, normal EXdi value is greater than 3.6 cm and 4.7 cm during a maximum inspiratory effort in women and in men, respectively. EXdi is poorly associated with Pdi in healthy subjects ($r = 0.44$; $p = 0.02$)[48] and with Ptr,stim in mechanically ventilated patients ($r = 0.45$, 95% CI 0.20 to 0.65, $p = 0.001$).[50] An EXdi lower than 1 cm is associated with weaning failure.[10] Interestingly, Spadaro et al. observed that the ratio of diaphragm excursion over respiratory rate (> 1.3 breaths/min/mm) was a better predictor of weaning outcome than the rapid shallow breathing index [AUC : 0.89 (0.76–0.95) < 0.0001, 0.72 (0.57–0.83) 0.011, respectively].[34] Other authors have attempted to integrate the EXdi with the inspiratory time, a variable called excursion-time index (product of diaphragm excursion and inspiratory time). The latter appears to be significantly lower in patients failing the weaning test compared to their counterparts (1.64 + 1.19 cm.s^{-1}, 2.42 + 1.55 cm.s^{-1}, respectively, $p < 0.03$). However, the performance of this test for predicting weaning success was quite modest (sensitivity of 79% and specificity of 75% to predict successful extubation).[49]

Ultrasound estimates of diaphragm thickness are correlated to direct anatomical measurements.[51] The lower limit of normal for diaphragm thickness has been reported to be 0.15 cm in healthy subjects with wide baseline range of values.[52] The reproducibility of diaphragm thickness as measured by ultrasound is good.[17, 51, 52] Diaphragm thickness is not correlated with marker of pressure generating capacity[50] and diaphragm thickness is not associated with weaning outcome.[50, 53, 54] A recent study conducted in patients with

67

amyotrophic lateral sclerosis did not find a correlation between histologically proven atrophy and the pressure generated capacity of the diaphragm.[55] Diaphragm ultrasound can detect decrease in thickness suggesting diaphragm atrophy[2, 17, 56, 57] but increase in thickness has also been reported while the significance of this observation remains unclear.[17] The significance of the diaphragm thickness remains unclear and should be considered with caution when estimating the function.

TFdi expresses the percentage of change in diaphragm thickness during its contraction. One study compared TFdi and Ptr,stim in mechanically ventilated patients and found that a cut-off value of TFdi < 29% was associated with diaphragm dysfunction.[50] Under pressure-support ventilation, a significant correlation was found between TFdi and Ptr,stim (rho = 0.87, p < 0.001), provided that patients trigger the ventilator.[50] There is no significant correlation between TFdi and Ptr,stim at initiation of mechanical ventilation, i.e., when inspiratory efforts are absent or insufficient.[50] The correlation between TFdi and diaphragm function is not univocal because the thickening is a one-dimension measurement whereas diaphragm contraction results from an active three-dimension displacement of muscle volume.[35] Therefore, the correlation between diaphragm thickening fraction and markers of pressure generating capacity is only moderate, ranging from $r^2 = 0.28$ in healthy subjects[17] to $r = 0.87$[50] and $r = 0.70$[58] in mechanically ventilated patients. This wide range indicates a limited validity of diaphragm thickening fraction to quantify diaphragm effort. A threshold of diaphragm thickening fraction < 29% has been associated with diaphragm dysfunction in patients under mechanical ventilation[50] and cut-off values for predicting successful extubation ranged from 25% to 35%.[36] However, in a series of patients who were extubated after a successful weaning trial, the TFdi was not significantly different in patients who succeeded in the extubation and those who failed (p = 0.67).[59] It may suggest that TFdi is not a discriminant variable to predict extubation outcome after a successful weaning trial.

Beyond standard technique, ultrasound derived indices are currently being investigated. Shear wave elastography (SWE) allows direct and real-time quantification of tissue stiffness. SWE measures non-invasively shear wave velocity, remotely generated, propagating in a target tissue.[60, 61] Shear wave velocity is directly correlated with tissue stiffness. In healthy subjects, shear modulus of the diaphragm (SMdi) displays a strong correlation with Pdi during both isovolumetric (R = 0.82, 95%) and inspiratory threshold loading effort (R = 0.70, 95%).[62] In mechanically ventilated patients, SMdi and Pdi global correlation was not as high (R = 0.45, p < 0.0001) as in healthy.[63] This may be explained by the smaller albeit more physiological range of Pdi. Tachypnea which, by reducing the inspiratory time, impairs the accuracy of SWE in measuring diaphragm stiffness at peak inspiration.

Tissue Doppler imaging is another ultrasound technique recently applied to the diaphragm.[64] Poulard et al. applied this technique in healthy subjects and reported that diaphragm maximal velocity was correlated with Pdi during a magnetic stimulation of the phrenic nerves in healthy subjects, r = 0.75 (p < 0.0001).[65] In the context of weaning, Soilemezi et al. reported that diaphragm peak contraction and relaxation velocity as obtained by tissue Doppler imaging were significantly lower in weaning failure patients as compared to successfully weaned patients.[66]

The speckle tracking technique is derived from the echocardiography and aims at analysing the longitudinal diaphragm shortening (strain).[67, 68] The correlation between TFdi and diaphragm strain is moderate (r^2 0.44, p < 0.001) whereas the correlation between diaphragm strain and diaphragm excursion is weak (r^2 0.14, p < 0.001).[68] By contrast, the correlation between strain and transdiaphragmatic pressure is high (r^2 0.72, (p < 0.0001).[67]

Electrical Activity of the Diaphragm

Diaphragm electrical activity can be measured by surface electromyography (EMG) or multi-array esophageal electrodes. The main advantage of surface EMG is that it is non-invasive, but it is frequently contaminated by the electrocardiogram or other muscles activity. Multi-array esophageal electrodes can facilitate the recording of the electrical activity of the diaphragm (EAdi) allowing continuous monitoring. Piquilloud et al. reported a broad range of median EAdi peaks in spontaneously breathing healthy subjects (from 5 μV to 30 μV)[69] which explains the large within-subject variability of EAdi derived indices.[70] Therefore, EAdi values are difficult to interpret, as only very limited data concerning "normal" values are currently available. However, it is interesting to combine EAdi with pressure-generated capacity indices to evaluate the neuromechanical coupling. A strong correlation has been reported between EAdi and Pdi, during end-expiratory occlusion, suggesting that the neuromechanical efficiency ratio (ΔPdi/ΔEAdi) could be useful to estimate inspiratory effort.[37] Lastly, the conversion of EAdi into V_T can also be studied by calculating the neuroventilatory efficiency index (V_T/EAdi). V_T/EAdi ratio can allow distinction between success or failure SBT patients at the beginning and during the weaning trial.[71]

Conclusion

The evaluation of the diaphragm function in mechanically ventilated patients may be useful to better understand the interactions between mechanical ventilation and patient's respiratory efforts. Ultrasound seems the perfect tool to achieve this ambition as it provides a direct and continuous evaluation of the diaphragm function. However, further efforts are needed to address technical limitations before generalizing the use of this tool as a reference technique. Theoretically, monitoring the diaphragm function could help to titrate the ventilatory support according to the patient's needs. The goal would be to prevent the risk of respiratory muscles disuse (over-assistance) and the risk of muscles injury (under-assistance).

Key points

Key point 1
There are several risk factors for diaphragm dysfunction: respiratory muscles disuse induced by mechanical ventilation, sepsis, shock states.

Key point 2
Diaphragm dysfunction is highly prevalent in mechanically ventilated patients: 63% of the patients at the time of admission, up to 80% of the patients at the time of prolonged weaning from mechanical ventilation.

Key point 3
The diaphragm function is estimated by the measurement of the transdiaphragmatic pressure (Pdi)
  Pdi = gastric pressure (Pga) – esophageal pressure (Pes)

Key point 4
Ultrasound evaluation of the diaphragm function:

Apposition zone: to estimate the diaphragm thickening fraction and diaphragm thickness

Subcostal approach: to estimate the diaphragm excursion

Key point 5
Assessment of the diaphragm function in mechanically ventilated patients
Underestimated prevalence of the disease, several risk factors

Physiological estimate: the transdiaphragmatic pressure

Standardized measurement with the bilateral anterior magnetic phrenic nerves stimulation

Diaphragm ultrasound: thickening fraction, excursion (to perform with the lower ventilator support to approach the diaphragm function)

References

1. Demoule A, Jung B, Prodanovic H, Diaphragm dysfunction on admission to the intensive care unit. Prevalence, risk factors, and prognostic impact-a prospective study. *Am J Respir Crit Care Med*. 2013;188(2):213–219. doi:10.1164/rccm.201209-1668OC

2. Goligher EC, Dres M, Fan E, et al. Mechanical ventilation-induced diaphragm atrophy strongly impacts clinical outcomes. *Am J Respir Crit Care Med*. 2018;197(2):204–213. doi:10.1164/rccm.201703-0536OC

3. Dres M, Demoule A. Monitoring diaphragm function in the ICU. *Curr Opin Crit Care*. 2020;26(1):18–25. doi:10.1097/MCC.0000000000000682

4. Dres M, Goligher EC, Heunks LMA, Brochard LJ. Critical illness-associated diaphragm weakness. *Intensive Care Med*. 2017;43(10):1441–1452. doi:10.1007/s00134-017-4928-4

5. Goligher EC, Laghi F, Detsky ME, et al. Measuring diaphragm thickness with ultrasound in mechanically ventilated patients: feasibility, reproducibility and validity. *Intensive Care Med*. 2015;41(4):734. doi:10.1007/s00134-015-3724-2

6. Sklar MC, Dres M, Fan E, et al. Association of low baseline diaphragm muscle mass with prolonged mechanical ventilation and mortality among critically Ill adults. *JAMA Netw Open*. 2020;3(2):e1921520. doi:10.1001/jamanetworkopen.2019.21520

7. Jaber S, Petrof BJ, Jung B, et al. Rapidly progressive diaphragmatic weakness and injury during mechanical ventilation in humans. *Am J Respir Crit Care Med*. 2011;183(3):364–371. doi:10.1164/rccm.201004-0670OC

8. Jung B, Moury PH, Mahul M, et al. Diaphragmatic dysfunction in patients with ICU-acquired weakness and its impact on extubation failure. *Intensive Care Med*. 2016;42(5):853–861. doi:10.1007/s00134-015-4125-2

9. Dres M, Dubé B-P, Mayaux J, et al. Coexistence and impact of limb muscle and diaphragm weakness at time of liberation from mechanical ventilation in medical intensive care unit patients. *Am J Respir Crit Care Med*. 2017;195(1):57–66. doi:10.1164/rccm.201602-0367OC

10. Kim WY, Suh HJ, Hong S-B, Koh Y, Lim C-M. Diaphragm dysfunction assessed by ultrasonography: influence on weaning from mechanical ventilation. *Crit Care Med*. 2011;39(12):2627–2630. doi:10.1097/CCM.0b013e3182266408

11. Hermans G, Agten A, Testelmans D, Decramer M, Gayan-Ramirez G. Increased duration of mechanical ventilation is associated with decreased diaphragmatic force: a prospective observational study. *Crit Care.* 2010;14(4):R127. doi:10.1186/cc9094

12. Le Bourdelles G, Viires N, Boczkowski J, Seta N, Pavlovic D, Aubier M. Effects of mechanical ventilation on diaphragmatic contractile properties in rats. *Am J Respir Crit Care Med.* 1994;149(6):1539–1544. doi:10.1164/ajrccm.149.6.8004310

13. Vassilakopoulos T, Petrof BJ. Ventilator-induced diaphragmatic dysfunction. *Am J Respir Crit Care Med.* 2004;169(3):336–341. doi:10.1164/rccm.200304-489CP

14. Sassoon CSH, Caiozzo VJ, Manka A, Sieck GC. Altered diaphragm contractile properties with controlled mechanical ventilation. *J Appl Physiol.* 2002;92(6):2585–2595. doi:10.1152/japplphysiol.01213.2001

15. Levine S, Nguyen T, Taylor N, et al. Rapid disuse atrophy of diaphragm fibers in mechanically ventilated humans. *N Engl J Med.* 2008;358(13):1327–1335. doi:10.1056/NEJMoa070447

16. Goligher EC, Brochard LJ, Reid WD, et al. Diaphragmatic myotrauma: a mediator of prolonged ventilation and poor patient outcomes in acute respiratory failure. *Lancet Respir Med.* 2019;7(1):90–98. doi:10.1016/S2213-2600(18)30366-7

17. Goligher EC, Fan E, Herridge MS, et al. Evolution of diaphragm thickness during mechanical ventilation. impact of inspiratory effort. *Am J Respir Crit Care Med.* 2015;192(9):1080–1088. doi:10.1164/rccm.201503-0620OC

18. Orozco-Levi M, Lloreta J, Minguella J, Serrano S, Broquetas JM, Gea J. Injury of the human diaphragm associated with exertion and chronic obstructive pulmonary disease. *Am J Respir Crit Care Med.* 2001;164(9):1734–1739. doi:10.1164/ajrccm.164.9.2011150

19. Demoule A, Molinari N, Jung B, et al. Patterns of diaphragm function in critically ill patients receiving prolonged mechanical ventilation: a prospective longitudinal study. *Ann Intensive Care.* 2016;6(1):75. doi:10.1186/s13613-016-0179-8

20. Dres M, Goligher EC, Dubé B-P, et al. Diaphragm function and weaning from mechanical ventilation: an ultrasound and phrenic nerve stimulation clinical study. *Ann Intensive Care.* 2018;8(1):53. doi:10.1186/s13613-018-0401-y

21. Manders E, Bonta PI, Kloek JJ, et al. Reduced force of diaphragm muscle fibers in patients with chronic thromboembolic pulmonary hypertension. *Am J Physiol Lung Cell Mol Physiol.* 2016;311(1):L20–28. doi:10.1152/ajplung.00113.2016

22. Kelley RC, Ferreira LF. Diaphragm abnormalities in heart failure and aging: mechanisms and integration of cardiovascular and respiratory pathophysiology. *Heart Fail Rev.* 2017;22(2):191–207. doi:10.1007/s10741-016-9549-4

23. Adler D, Dupuis-Lozeron E, Richard J-C, Janssens J-P, Brochard L. Does inspiratory muscle dysfunction predict readmission after intensive care unit discharge? *Am J Respir Crit Care Med.* 2014;190(3):347–350. doi:10.1164/rccm.201404-0655LE

24. Medrinal C, Prieur G, Frenoy É, et al. Respiratory weakness after mechanical ventilation is associated with one-year mortality: a prospective study. *Crit Care.* 2016;20(1):231. doi:10.1186/s13054-016-1418-y

25. Saccheri C, Morawiec E, Delemazure J, et al. ICU-acquired weakness, diaphragm dysfunction and long-term outcomes of critically ill patients. *Ann Intensive Care.* 2020;10(1):1. doi:10.1186/s13613-019-0618-4

26. Marchioni A, Castaniere I, Tonelli R, et al. Ultrasound-assessed diaphragmatic impairment is a predictor of outcomes in patients with acute exacerbation of chronic obstructive pulmonary disease undergoing noninvasive ventilation. *Crit Care.* 2018;22(1):109. doi:10.1186/s13054-018-2033-x

27. Goligher EC, Dres M, Patel BK, et al. Lung- and diaphragm-protective ventilation. *Am J Respir Crit Care Med.* 2020;202(7):950–961. doi:10.1164/rccm.202003-0655CP

28. Goligher EC, Jonkman AH, Dianti J, et al. Clinical strategies for implementing lung and diaphragm-protective ventilation: avoiding insufficient and excessive effort. *Intensive Care Med.* 2020;46(12):2314–2326. doi:10.1007/s00134-020-06288-9

29. Boles J-M, Bion J, Connors A, et al. Weaning from mechanical ventilation. *Eur Respir J.* 2007;29(5):1033–1056. doi:10.1183/09031936.00010206

30. McConville JF, Kress JP. Weaning patients from the ventilator. *N Engl J Med.* 2012;367(23):2233–2239. doi:10.1056/NEJMra1203367

31. De Jonghe B, Bastuji-Garin S, Durand M-C, et al. Respiratory weakness is associated with limb weakness and delayed weaning in critical illness. *Crit Care Med.* 2007;35(9):2007–2015.

32. Garnacho-Montero J, Amaya-Villar R, García-Garmendía JL, Madrazo-Osuna J, Ortiz-Leyba C. Effect of critical illness polyneuropathy on the withdrawal from mechanical ventilation and the length of stay in septic patients. *Crit Care Med.* 2005;33(2):349–354. doi:10.1097/01.ccm.0000153521.41848.7e

33. Lerolle N, Guérot E, Dimassi S, et al. Ultrasonographic diagnostic criterion for severe diaphragmatic dysfunction after cardiac surgery. *Chest.* 2009;135(2):401–407. doi:10.1378/chest.08-1531

34. Spadaro S, Grasso S, Dres M, et al. Point of care ultrasound to identify diaphragmatic dysfunction after thoracic surgery. *Anesthesiology.* Published online May 22, 2019. doi:10.1097/ALN.0000000000002774

35. Laveneziana P, Albuquerque A, Aliverti A, et al. ERS statement on respiratory muscle testing at rest and during exercise. *Eur Respir J.* Published online April 7, 2019. doi:10.1183/13993003.01214-2018

36. Dres M, Demoule A. Diaphragm dysfunction during weaning from mechanical ventilation: an underestimated phenomenon with clinical implications. *Crit Care.* 2018;22:73. doi:10.1186/s13054-018-1992-2

37. Bellani G, Bronco A, Arrigoni Marocco S, et al. Measurement of diaphragmatic electrical activity by surface electromyography in intubated subjects and its relationship with inspiratory effort. *Respir Care.* 2018;63(11):1341–1349. doi:10.4187/respcare.06176

38. Black LF, Hyatt RE. Maximal respiratory pressures: normal values and relationship to age and sex. *Am Rev Respir Dis.* 1969;99(5):696–702. doi:10.1164/arrd.1969.99.5.696

39. Caruso P, Friedrich C, Denari SD, Ruiz SA, Deheinzelin D. The unidirectional valve is the best method to determine maximal inspiratory pressure during weaning. *Chest.* 1999;115(4):1096–1101.

40. Multz AS, Aldrich TK, Prezant DJ, Karpel JP, Hendler JM. Maximal inspiratory pressure is not a reliable test of inspiratory muscle strength in mechanically ventilated patients. *Am Rev Respir Dis.* 1990;142(3):529–532. doi:10.1164/ajrccm/142.3.529

41. Watson AC, Hughes PD, Louise Harris M, et al. Measurement of twitch transdiaphragmatic, esophageal, and endotracheal tube pressure with bilateral anterolateral magnetic phrenic nerve stimulation in patients in the intensive care unit. *Crit Care Med.* 2001;29(7):1325–1331.

42. Sahn SA, Lakshminarayan S. Bedside criteria for discontinuation of mechanical ventilation. *Chest.* 1973;63(6):1002–1005. doi:10.1378/chest.63.6.1002

43. Akoumianaki E, Maggiore SM, Valenza F, et al. The application of esophageal pressure measurement in patients with respiratory failure. *Am J Respir Crit Care Med.* 2014;189(5):520–531. doi:10.1164/rccm.201312-2193CI

44. Zambon M, Greco M, Bocchino S, Cabrini L, Beccaria PF, Zangrillo A. Assessment of diaphragmatic dysfunction in the critically ill patient with ultrasound: a systematic review. *Intensive Care Med.* 2017;43(1):29–38. doi:10.1007/s00134-016-4524-z

45. Vetrugno L, Guadagnin GM, Barbariol F, Langiano N, Zangrillo A, Bove T. Ultrasound imaging for diaphragm dysfunction: a narrative literature review. *J Cardiothorac Vasc Anesth.* Published online January 4, 2019. doi:10.1053/j.jvca.2019.01.003

46. Tuinman PR, Jonkman AH, Dres M, et al. Respiratory muscle ultrasonography: methodology, basic and advanced principles and clinical applications in ICU and ED patients-a narrative review. *Intensive Care Med.* 2020;46(4):594–605. doi:10.1007/s00134-019-05892-8

47. Boussuges A, Gole Y, Blanc P. Diaphragmatic motion studied by m-mode ultrasonography: methods, reproducibility, and normal values. *Chest.* 2009;135(2):391–400. doi:10.1378/chest.08-1541

48. Spiesshoefer J, Henke C, Herkenrath SD, et al. Noninvasive prediction of twitch transdiaphragmatic pressure: insights from spirometry, diaphragm ultrasound, and phrenic nerve stimulation studies. *Respiration.* 2019;98(4):301–311. doi:10.1159/000501171

49. Palkar A, Narasimhan M, Greenberg H, et al. Diaphragm excursion-time index: a new parameter using ultrasonography to predict extubation outcome. *Chest.* 2018;153(5):1213–1220. doi:10.1016/j.chest.2018.01.007

50. Dubé B-P, Dres M, Mayaux J, Demiri S, Similowski T, Demoule A. Ultrasound evaluation of diaphragm function in mechanically ventilated patients: comparison to phrenic stimulation and prognostic implications. *Thorax.* 2017;72(9):811–818. doi:10.1136/thoraxjnl-2016-209459

51. Wait JL, Nahormek PA, Yost WT, Rochester DP. Diaphragmatic thickness-lung volume relationship in vivo. *J Appl Physiol.* 1989;67(4):1560–1568. doi:10.1152/jappl.1989.67.4.1560

52. Boon AJ, Harper CJ, Ghahfarokhi LS, Strommen JA, Watson JC, Sorenson EJ. Two-dimensional ultrasound imaging of the diaphragm: quantitative values in normal subjects. *Muscle Nerve*. 2013;47(6):884–889. doi:10.1002/mus.23702

53. Ferrari G, De Filippi G, Elia F, Panero F, Volpicelli G, Aprà F. Diaphragm ultrasound as a new index of discontinuation from mechanical ventilation. *Crit Ultrasound J*. 2014;6(1):8. doi:10.1186/2036-7902-6-8

54. DiNino E, Gartman EJ, Sethi JM, McCool FD. Diaphragm ultrasound as a predictor of successful extubation from mechanical ventilation. *Thorax*. 2014;69(5):423–427. doi:10.1136/thoraxjnl-2013-204111

55. Guimarães-Costa R, Similowski T, Rivals I, et al. Human diaphragm atrophy in amyotrophic lateral sclerosis is not predicted by routine respiratory measures. *Eur Respir J*. 2019;53(2):1801749. doi:10.1183/13993003.01749-2018

56. Grosu HB, Lee YI, Lee J, Eden E, Eikermann M, Rose KM. Diaphragm muscle thinning in patients who are mechanically ventilated. *Chest*. 2012;142(6):1455–1460. doi:10.1378/chest.11-1638

57. Schepens T, Verbrugghe W, Dams K, Corthouts B, Parizel PM, Jorens PG. The course of diaphragm atrophy in ventilated patients assessed with ultrasound: a longitudinal cohort study. *Crit Care*. 2015;19:422. doi:10.1186/s13054-015-1141-0

58. Umbrello M, Formenti P, Longhi D, et al. Diaphragm ultrasound as indicator of respiratory effort in critically ill patients undergoing assisted mechanical ventilation: a pilot clinical study. *Crit Care*. 2015;19:161. doi:10.1186/s13054-015-0894-9

59. Vivier E, Muller M, Putegnat J-B, et al. Inability of diaphragm ultrasound to predict extubation failure: a multicenter study. *Chest*. 2019;155(6):1131–1139. doi:10.1016/j.chest.2019.03.004

60. Deffieux T, Gennisson J-L, Bousquet L, et al. Investigating liver stiffness and viscosity for fibrosis, steatosis and activity staging using shear wave elastography. *J Hepatol*. 2015;62(2):317–324. doi:10.1016/j.jhep.2014.09.020

61. Chino K, Ohya T, Katayama K, Suzuki Y. Diaphragmatic shear modulus at various submaximal inspiratory mouth pressure levels. *Respir Physiol Neurobiol*. Published online March 19, 2018. doi:10.1016/j.resp.2018.03.009

62. Bachasson D, Dres M, Niérat M-C, et al. Diaphragm shear modulus reflects transdiaphragmatic pressure during isovolumetric inspiratory efforts and ventilation against inspiratory loading. *J Appl Physiol*. Published online February 7, 2019. doi:10.1152/japplphysiol.01060.2018

63. Fossé Q, Poulard T, Niérat M-C, et al. Ultrasound shear wave elastography for assessing diaphragm function in mechanically ventilated patients: a breath-by-breath analysis. *Crit Care*. 2020;24(1):669. doi:10.1186/s13054-020-03338-y

64. Cammarota G, Boniolo E, Tarquini R, Vaschetto R. Diaphragmatic excursion tissue Doppler sonographic assessment. *Intensive Care Med*. 2020;46(9):1759–1760. doi:10.1007/s00134-020-06015-4

65. Poulard T, Dres M, Niérat M-C, et al. Ultrafast ultrasound coupled with cervical magnetic stimulation for non-invasive and non-volitional assessment of diaphragm contractility. *J Physiol*. 2020;598(24):5627–5638. doi:10.1113/JP280457

66. Soilemezi E, Savvidou S, Sotiriou P, Smyrniotis D, Tsagourias M, Matamis D. Tissue Doppler Imaging of the Diaphragm in Healthy Subjects and Critically Ill Patients. *Am J Respir Crit Care Med*. 2020;202(7):1005–1012. doi:10.1164/rccm.201912-2341OC

67. Oppersma E, Hatam N, Doorduin J, et al. Functional assessment of the diaphragm by speckle tracking ultrasound during inspiratory loading. *J Appl Physiol*. 2017;123(5):1063–1070. doi:10.1152/japplphysiol.00095.2017

68. Orde SR, Boon AJ, Firth DG, Villarraga HR, Sekiguchi H. Diaphragm assessment by two dimensional speckle tracking imaging in normal subjects. *BMC Anesthesiol*. 2016;16(1):43. doi:10.1186/s12871-016-0201-6

69. Piquilloud L, Beloncle F, Richard J-CM, Mancebo J, Mercat A, Brochard L. Information conveyed by electrical diaphragmatic activity during unstressed, stressed and assisted spontaneous breathing: a physiological study. *Ann Intensive Care*. 2019;9(1):89. doi:10.1186/s13613-019-0564-1

70. Jansen D, Jonkman AH, Roesthuis L, et al. Estimation of the diaphragm neuromuscular efficiency index in mechanically ventilated critically ill patients. *Crit Care*. 2018;22(1):238. doi:10.1186/s13054-018-2172-0

71. Dres M, Schmidt M, Ferre A, Mayaux J, Similowski T, Demoule A. Diaphragm electromyographic activity as a predictor of weaning failure. *Intensive Care Med*. 2012;38(12):2017–2025. doi:10.1007/s00134-012-2700-3

7

Diaphragm Ultrasound during Weaning from Mechanical Ventilation

**Mark E. Haaksma, Heder J. de Vries,
Leo Heunks, and Pieter R. Tuinman**

DOI: 10.1201/9781003128694-10

Introduction

Weaning patients from mechanical ventilation is a daily, yet challenging part of intensive care medicine and has a large impact on patient outcome and intensive care unit (ICU) resources (1). The pathophysiology of weaning is complex and involves different organ systems including the lungs, heart, and respiratory muscles (2). In this regard, the role of the diaphragm has been the focus of recent research and its ultrasonographic evaluation has already become a popular application. Assessment of diaphragm excursion, tracking its thickness over time, and measuring the percentual change in thickness during a respiratory cycle opens up the possibilities to evaluate patient ventilator interaction, map atrophy, and determine its functional status (3–5). In this chapter, we discuss these and other subjects and highlight the most relevant points of diaphragm ultrasound when weaning patients from mechanical ventilation.

Ultrasound during Mechanical Ventilation

In healthy, spontaneously breathing people, contraction and with that caudal displacement of the diaphragm, is a direct indicator of its function. For mechanically ventilated patients, this issue becomes more complex due to the positive pressure delivered during inspiration by the ventilator (3, 6). Therefore, one should carefully consider three relevant components when assessing the diaphragm through ultrasound in ventilated patients: inspiratory pressure, PEEP (positive end expiratory pressure), and ventilator mode.

Inspiratory Pressure

The amount of positive pressure provided during inspiration by the ventilator can be viewed as the amount of assistance the diaphragm receives to generate an inspiratory effort. Increasing this pressure thus decreases the work the diaphragm needs to deliver and with that also its contractile activity (7, 8). As logically follows, this impacts the biometric data we obtain when assessing the diaphragm with ultrasound.

For example, when assessing thickness and thickening fraction, one has to realize that due to the assistance provided by the ventilator, the diaphragm will have to generate less effort and thus contractile activity will be reduced. This could result in a lower end inspiratory thickness and with that also in a lower thickening fraction. As follows, a decrease in, for example, thickening fraction does not necessarily have to indicate dysfunction, but could be a result of reduced activity. The same should also be considered when assessing diaphragm excursion, as this is at least equally, potentially even more strongly, influenced by ventilator assistance (9).

Additionally, in both instances (thickening fraction and excursion) one should consider that the pressure delivered by the ventilator also causes passive displacement of the diaphragm, which can't be distinguished from active displacement. This obviously affects interpretation of excursion measurement as both the active contraction and passive displacement work in the same direction (caudal displacement of the diaphragm), but also the thickening fraction to some extent. One can visualize the latter by passive flexion of the biceps muscle, which then also undergoes an increase in thickness.

In summary, with inspiratory assistance the use of excursion measurements is not recommended while use of the thickening fraction is possible, but limited.

Positive End Expiratory Pressure

Positive end expiratory pressure is an important factor during ultrasonographic assessment of the diaphragm. With the increase in end-expiratory lung volume, the diaphragm is flattened and shortened, as it can't reach its "normal" resting position at the end of expiration (10), thereby (potentially) limiting the range of motion available to the diaphragm. However, not only excursion but also diaphragm thickness is influenced by PEEP. For the sake of simplicity, the lower resting position can be viewed as passive-displacement, which, similar to the mechanism described above, results in an increased end-expiratory thickness (11). As such, this is not only an important consideration when tracking diaphragm atrophy over time, but also when assessing the functional status of the diaphragm through thickening fraction. The latter is impacted by an increased end-expiratory thickness which in turn potentially decreases the percentage change during a respiratory cycle.

Modes of Ventilation

Given the heterogeneity in ventilator modes, nomenclature, and accompanying sedation protocols, it is just as difficult to provide detailed information for each situation, as it is to give general recommendations. The critical consideration one should make is whether active diaphragm contraction is possible/present.

In mandatory modes of ventilation, as the name implies, the ventilator dictates the patient's respiration. These modes are typically used concomitantly with sedation, which reduces or potentially negates diaphragm activity. In these cases, any statements about diaphragm functionality are of little or no information. On the contrary, thickness measurements to track atrophy are still useful, with the caveats stated in the paragraphs above.

In assisted modes of ventilation, with certain exceptions such as triggering with accessory muscles or auto-triggering, one can generally assume there to be at least some degree of diaphragm activity. Nevertheless, one should consider that with very high levels of support activity inevitably decreases. At some point, this might even mimic a mandatory mode in terms of ultrasonographic assessment of the diaphragm.

Summary of Ultrasound in Mechanical Ventilation

During mechanical ventilation, ultrasonographic assessment of the diaphragm is valuable yet also challenging. The pressures delivered by the ventilator create important limitations by altering the diaphragm's resting position, range of motion, and effort delivered. Reference values for assessing diaphragm function under various ventilator settings are lacking. This should, however, not deter the clinician to use this valuable tool but to proceed with described caveats in mind. A summary is provided in Table 7.1.

Patient–Ventilator Interactions

Optimal patient–ventilator interaction is an important aspect of assisted ventilation and can be seen as an adequate response of the ventilator to the patient's inspiratory and

Table 7.1 Effects of mechanical ventilation on diaphragm ultrasound measurements

	Positive pressure	PEEP	Mode
Excursion	Active and passive displacement can't be distinguished	Caudal displacement, potentially decreased excursion	In controlled mode little/no active excursion
Thickness	Decreased end-inspiratory thickness	Increased end-expiratory thickness	n.a.
Thickening	Decreased end-inspiratory thickness	Increased end-expiratory thickness	In controlled mode little/no active thickening

expiratory needs. Patient–ventilator asynchrony is a common problem occurring in up to half of all mechanically ventilated patients and is associated with worse outcomes (12). Ultrasonographic evaluation of the diaphragm might be a valuable tool to elucidate the nature of the asynchrony (4). In the following section, we briefly describe this methodology. A summary is provided in Table 7.2. For an in-depth discussion of asynchronies we refer the reader to a recent review article (13).

Ineffective Triggering or Wasted Effort

Ineffective triggering or wasted efforts are caused by inadequate (i.e., too low) sensitivity of the ventilator to the patient's inspiratory signals. This can be detected by visualizing diaphragm motion or an increase in thickness without triggering of the ventilator.

Auto-triggering

Auto-triggering occurs when, due to inappropriate (i.e., too high) sensitivity of the ventilator, a breath is triggered in the absence of a patient's derived inspiratory signal. This can be detected by the lack of initial diaphragm motion or increase in thickness when the ventilator is triggered.

Trigger Delay

A trigger delay can, for example, occur when the threshold of the ventilator to trigger a breath is set too high. This can be detected by an initial excursion or thickening fraction of the diaphragm which is only later accompanied by a rise in airway pressure delivered by ventilator. This requires excessive and potentially harmful patient effort.

Double Trigger

Double triggering may occur if ventilator's inspiratory time falls short in comparison to the patient's inspiratory time. This can be detected by a steady increase in diaphragm motion or thickness during a single inspiration, which, however, triggers the ventilator twice within this inspiration, resulting in unwanted large tidal volumes.

Table 7.2 Summary of patient–ventilator asynchronies with their pressure waveforms and ultrasound correlate

Asynchrony	Explanation	Figure
Wasted effort	Ventilator not triggered despite diaphragm excursion	
Auto-triggering	Ventilator triggered without diaphragm thickening	
Trigger delay	Ventilator triggered with delay	
Double trigger	Ventilator triggered twice within one breath	
Reverse triggering	Ventilator triggered twice due to active excursion after passive displacement	

Upper curve is the pressure waveform; lower curve is excursion of the diaphragm visualized by ultrasound in M-mode.

Reverse Triggering

Reverse triggering can occur in sedated patients, which is hypothesized to result from stimulation of the respiratory control centres by passive mechanical insufflation of the thorax (14). As a consequence, after a mandatory breath delivered by the ventilator another breath is triggered by the patient instead of the machine. This can be detected by an active movement of the diaphragm after passive displacement which results in a higher excursion amplitude and creates a notch in the inspiratory excursion curve.

Diaphragm Ultrasound to Track Atrophy

Ultrasound offers the possibility to measure diaphragm thickness in the zone of apposition, as discussed in Chapter 4. Given its bedside availability and low patient burden, thickness measurements can be repeated on a daily basis to map the evolution of thickness over time.

Tracking diaphragm thickness is especially interesting in mechanically ventilated patients, as the reduction of contractile activity due to ventilator assistance is associated with diaphragm atrophy (8). This occurs at an alarmingly fast pace, with up to 57% decrease in muscle fibre cross-sectional area within three days of mechanical ventilation (15).

As a clinician, being aware of this is important, as evidence suggests that ultrasonographically assessed atrophy, i.e., reduction in thickness, of more than 10% from baseline is associated with a lower daily probability of being liberated from the ventilator and prolonged ICU admission (16).

Tracking atrophy thus opens up the possibility to identify patients at risk for longer ventilation and initiate timely intervention, i.e., diaphragm protective ventilation. This entails titrating ventilator support to stimulate adequate diaphragm contractility and potentially limit atrophy. It is discussed in more detail in the next section.

Diaphragm Ultrasound to Titrate Ventilator Settings

Titrating ventilator settings on the basis of diaphragm ultrasound is still largely uncharted territory. The underlying idea is to create "diaphragm protective ventilation", i.e., prevent over- or under-assistance by the ventilator which would respectively cause disuse atrophy and load-induced injury of the diaphragm (2, 17, 18). While this might seem trivial, studies have shown that loss of diaphragm thickness and functionality is associated with worse outcomes in ICU patients (16).

Diaphragm Ultrasound and Diaphragm Effort

The first hurdle that stills needs to be overcome is to find a feasible ultrasonographic approach that accurately reflects diaphragm effort. Thickening fraction would be the first thing that comes to mind, where a high value would reflect excessive effort and vice versa. Unfortunately, no clear cut-offs for "excessive" and "insufficient" effort have been elucidated so far, as normal ranges also vary strongly (19). To add insult to injury, a set amount of thickening fraction does not necessarily have to correlate with a set amount of effort. In this regard, several studies have evaluated change of thickening fraction depending on the amount of assistance provided and determined its correlation to a measure of effort (7, 9). While these studies showed promising results, they were conducted in small groups and a large range of effort could be associated with a set thickening fraction (20).

Additionally, if this problem is overcome, one still needs to consider the combination of diaphragm and lung protective ventilation (18). While these are definitely not mutually exclusive, they are also not necessarily complementary to each other. For example, a common situation might be the necessity to sedate and even paralyze a patient's diaphragm to ensure protective pulmonary pressures, which, however, comes at the cost of decreasing or eliminating diaphragm activity.

In Clinical Practice

While seemingly difficult to apply in clinical practice, there are possibilities to do so. A recent observational study identified that a thickening fraction between 15% and 30% is associated with shortest duration of mechanical ventilation (16). Practically speaking, one could thus titrate the ventilator assist to let thickening fraction fall within this range, ideally without sacrificing respiratory parameters such as tidal volume and respiratory rate (4, 16, 18).

A Comprehensive Ultrasound Approach during Weaning from Mechanical Ventilation: Ultrasound of Diaphragm, Heart, and Lungs

Weaning from the ventilator can be considered as a cardio-pulmonary stress test and requires complex interaction and adaptation of diaphragm, heart, and lungs. As such, optimization of respiratory muscle-, pulmonary-, and cardiac function is essential. Ultrasound offers the unique possibility to monitor all these organ systems and potential changes repeatedly through the course of weaning and as a diagnostic tool in case of failed attempts (2, 4, 21). With this idea in mind, a recent review highlighted a simple holistic ultrasound approach to weaning: the "ABCD-approach" (4).

ABCD-Approach

The ABCD-approach is a simple standardization for a holistic ultrasound approach when evaluating the weaning patient. Each letter refers to the evaluation of the organ system relevant in the weaning process.

A) Aeration score and pleural effusion: lung aeration is evaluated according to previously published protocols. An aeration score of > 17 or an increase of more than six B-lines (vertical comet-tail artefact) during a spontaneous breathing trial is associated with failed extubation (22,23). Additionally, the presence, extent, and nature of pleural effusion is determined.

B) Below the diaphragm: the presence of ascites or abdominal abscesses is evaluated, as they could potentially have a detrimental effect on respiratory mechanics.

C) Cardiac: cardiac function is evaluated. The extent is dependent on proficiency of the clinician. Simpler approaches include gauging left ventricular function by eyeballing or measurement of tricuspid annular plane systolic excursion (TAPSE) for right ventricular function. In more experienced hands, the velocity time index or the E/A-ratio can be calculated to determine diastolic function.

D) Diaphragm: diaphragm thickening fraction and excursion are evaluated as described in Chapters 3 and 4 of this book. Low values for thickening fraction and excursion are associated with extubation failure (see below).

E) Extra-diaphragmatic respiratory muscles: activation, i.e., thickening, of the lateral abdominal muscles and the parasternal intercostal muscles is evaluated as described in Chapter 11 of this book. Activation of the muscles is indicative of a higher work of breathing or low diaphragm capacity (2, 24).

In Clinical Practice

As of yet, there are no trials evaluating the benefit of implementing such an approach in clinical practice. Nevertheless, it offers a simple method of charting factors influencing the weaning process. It can be applied at early stages to identify possibilities for optimization of cardio-respiratory function or as a diagnostic tool after a failed extubation attempt.

Ultrasound to Predict Extubation Success/Failure

Deciding to extubate the patient remains a daunting task for any intensivist, given the severe consequences associated with failed attempts (1). As such, the search for tools to aid the clinician in this task continues, with ultrasonographic assessment of the diaphragm being one of the latest additions. The underlying hypothesis is that the diaphragm, as the main driving force of respiration, plays a crucial role in transitioning from mechanical ventilation to spontaneous breathing. In the next section, we describe the potential application of diaphragm ultrasound to predict extubation outcome in clinical practice and discuss its limitations.

Thickening Fraction

Thickening fraction of the diaphragm is the most researched index as predictor of extubation outcome. Values above 30–36% have been identified as the threshold to predict a successful outcome with highest diagnostic accuracy (25–27). However, more recently studies have shown conflicting results demonstrating that diaphragm ultrasound might not be as good a predictor as previously believed (28, 29).

If a closer look at available evidence is made, it quickly becomes apparent that studies are hardly comparable to each other. Study populations, ventilator settings (i.e., inspiratory pressure, PEEP, etc.) at the time of ultrasound measurements and the definition of extubation failure vary strongly. These discrepancies require new studies with standardized protocols and randomized trials before definitive conclusions can be drawn about thickening fraction as predictor of extubation failure. Until then, using thickening fraction as an independent predictor of extubation outcome can't be recommended.

Excursion

Diaphragm excursion is a less frequently used parameter for predicting extubation outcome. Nevertheless, several studies have evaluated its use and a recent meta-analysis demonstrated it having substantial diagnostic accuracy to predict a successful outcome (30). The question then remains why it hasn't gained popularity thus far. The answer to this is the high variation in cut-offs determined by various studies. In the previously mentioned meta-analysis alone, these ranged from 1 to 2.7cm. In addition, there is evidence that excursion for a fixed lung volume also strongly differs according to body positioning (31). Furthermore, as for thickening fraction, the same problem of a large heterogeneity in study design exists.

Recently, a study evaluated the incorporation of diaphragm excursion to the well-known rapid shallow breathing index (32). While the study showed promising results, this approach still needs to be validated in larger trials.

As for now, also for diaphragm excursion it has to be concluded that it can't be used as an independent predictor of extubation outcome.

Table 7.3 Potential applications of diaphragm ultrasound during the weaning phase

	Asynchrony	Diaphragm protective ventilation	Predict extubation outcome	Diagnostic tool
Excursion	Wasted effort, trigger delay	Double trigger, reverse triggering	Excursion > 1–2.5 cm associated with success	Diaphragm dysfunction and paralysis
Thickness		Identify ventilator over-assist through diaphragm atrophy		Diaphragm atrophy
Thickening	Auto-triggering	Titrate ventilator settings for diaphragm protective ventilation	Thickening fraction > 30–36% associated with success	Diaphragm dysfunction and paralysis

In Clinical Practice

Overall, the aforementioned limitations of discussed approaches seemingly provide a limited role of diaphragm ultrasound in predicting extubation outcome. A key step will be to determine in which subgroups and under which conditions it can act as a reliable predictor. Until then, the role of diaphragm ultrasound should be reserved for diagnosing diaphragm weakness in difficult to wean patients.

Chapter Summary

In this chapter, we outlined the most important aspects of diaphragm ultrasound during mechanical ventilation, especially in the weaning phase. If the limitations as consequence of ventilator assistance are kept in mind, it is a useful and versatile tool that can provide the clinician with vital information about the differential diagnosis of difficult weaning or failed extubation and potentially aid in synchronizing patient–ventilator interaction (Table 7.3).

References

1. Béduneau G, Pham T, Schortgen F, Piquilloud L, Zogheib E, Jonas M, et al. Epidemiology of weaning outcome according to a new definition. The WIND study. *Am J Respir Crit Care Med*. 2017 Mar 15;195(6):772–83.

2. Haaksma ME, Tuinman PR, Heunks L. Weaning the patient: between protocols and physiology. *Curr Opin Crit Care*. 2021 Feb;27(1):29–36.

3. Haaksma ME, Atmowihardjo L, Heunks L, Spoelstra-de Man A, Tuinman PR. Ultrasound imaging of the diaphragm: facts and future. A guide for the bedside clinician. *Neth J Crit Care*. 2018;26(2):6.

4. Tuinman PR, Jonkman AH, Dres M, Shi Z-H, Goligher EC, Goffi A, et al. Respiratory muscle ultrasonography: methodology, basic and advanced principles and clinical applications in ICU and ED patients: a narrative review. *Intensive Care Med.* 2020 Jan 14;46(4):594–605.

5. Zambon M, Greco M, Bocchino S, Cabrini L, Beccaria PF, Zangrillo A. Assessment of diaphragmatic dysfunction in the critically ill patient with ultrasound: a systematic review. *Intensive Care Med* [Internet]. 2016; Available from: http://link.springer.com/10.1007/s00134-016-4524-z

6. Matamis D, Soilemezi E, Tsagourias M, Akoumianaki E, Dimassi S, Boroli F, et al. Sonographic evaluation of the diaphragm in critically ill patients. Technique and clinical applications. *Intensive Care Med.* 2013;39(5):801–10.

7. Vivier E, Dessap AM, Dimassi S, Vargas F, Lyazidi A, Thille AW, et al. Diaphragm ultrasonography to estimate the work of breathing during non-invasive ventilation. *Intensive Care Med.* 2012;38(5):796–803.

8. Goligher EC, Fan E, Herridge MS, Murray A, Vorona S, Brace D, et al. Evolution of diaphragm thickness during mechanical ventilation: Impact of inspiratory effort. *Am J Respir Crit Care Med.* 2015;192(9):1080–8.

9. Umbrello M, Formenti P, Longhi D, Galimberti A, Piva I, Pezzi A, et al. Diaphragm ultrasound as indicator of respiratory effort in critically ill patients undergoing assisted mechanical ventilation: a pilot clinical study. *Crit Care Lond Engl.* 2015;19(1):161.

10. Lindqvist J, van den Berg M, van der Pijl R, Hooijman PE, Beishuizen A, Elshof J, et al. Positive end-expiratory pressure ventilation induces longitudinal atrophy in diaphragm fibers. *Am J Respir Crit Care Med.* 2018 Aug 15;198(4):472–85.

11. Jansen D, Jonkman AH, De Vries HJ, Marcus JT, Ottenheijm CAC, Heunks LMA. Late breaking abstract - positive end-expiratory pressure affects geometry and function of the human diaphragm. *Eur Respir J.* 2020 Sep 7;56(suppl 64):3719.

12. Vaporidi K, Babalis D, Chytas A, Lilitsis E, Kondili E, Amargianitakis V, et al. Clusters of ineffective efforts during mechanical ventilation: impact on outcome. *Intensive Care Med.* 2017 Feb;43(2):184–91.

13. Mirabella L, Cinnella G, Costa R, Cortegiani A, Tullo L, Rauseo M, et al. Patient-ventilator asynchronies: clinical implications and practical solutions. *Respir Care.* 2020 Nov;65(11):1751–66.

14. de Vries HJ, Jonkman AH, Tuinman PR, Girbes ARJ, Heunks LMA. Respiratory entrainment and reverse triggering in a mechanically ventilated patient. *Ann Am Thorac Soc.* 2019 Apr;16(4):499–505.

15. Levine S, Nguyen T, Taylor N, Friscia ME, Budak MT, Rothenberg P, et al. Rapid disuse atrophy of diaphragm fibers in mechanically ventilated humans. *New Engl J Med* 2008;358(13):1327–35.

16. Goligher EC, Dres M, Fan E, Rubenfeld GD, Scales DC, Herridge MS, et al. Mechanical ventilation–induced diaphragm atrophy strongly impacts clinical outcomes. *Am J Respir Crit Care Med.* 2018 Jan 15;197(2):204–13.

17. Zambon M, Beccaria P, Matsuno J, Gemma M, Frati E, Colombo S, et al. Mechanical ventilation and diaphragmatic atrophy in critically Ill patients: an ultrasound study. *Crit Care Med.* 2016 Jul;44(7):1347–52.

18. Goligher EC, Dres M, Patel BK, Sahetya SK, Beitler JR, Telias I, et al. Lung and diaphragm-protective ventilation. *Am J Respir Crit Care Med*. 2020;202(7):950-961.

19. Seok JI, Kim SY, Walker FO, Kwak SG, Kwon DH. Ultrasonographic findings of the normal diaphragm: thickness and contractility. *Ann Clin Neurophysiol*. 2017;19(2):131.

20. Haaksma M, Tuinman PR, Heunks L. Ultrasound to assess diaphragmatic function in the critically ill: a critical perspective. *Ann Transl Med*. 2017 Mar;5(5):114–114.

21. Doorduin J, van der Hoeven JG, Heunks LMA. The differential diagnosis for failure to wean from mechanical ventilation: *Curr Opin Anaesthesiol*. 2016 Apr;29(2):150–7.

22. Ferré A, Guillot M, Lichtenstein D, Mezière G, Richard C, Teboul J-L, et al. Lung ultrasound allows the diagnosis of weaning-induced pulmonary oedema. *Intensive Care Med*. 2019 May;45(5):601–8.

23. Soummer A, Perbet S, Brisson H, Arbelot C, Constantin J-M, Lu Q, et al. Ultrasound assessment of lung aeration loss during a successful weaning trial predicts postextubation distress*: *Crit Care Med*. 2012 Jul;40(7):2064–72.

24. Dres M, Dubé B-P, Goligher E, Vorona S, Demiri S, Morawiec E, et al. Usefulness of parasternal intercostal muscle ultrasound during weaning from mechanical ventilation. *Anesthesiology*. 2020 May;132(5):1114–25.

25. DiNino E, Gartman EJ, Sethi JM, McCool FD. Diaphragm ultrasound as a predictor of successful extubation from mechanical ventilation. *Thorax*. 2014;69(5):423–7.

26. Govanni Ferrari GDF, Fabrizio Elia1, Francesco Panero GV and FA. Diaphragm ultrasound as a new index of discontinuation from mechanical ventilation. *Thorax*. 2014;69(5):431–5.

27. Farghaly S, Hasan AA. Diaphragm ultrasound as a new method to predict extubation outcome in mechanically ventilated patients. *Aust Crit Care Off J Confed Aust Crit Care Nurses*. 2016 Apr 21;30(1):37–43.

28. Vivier E, Muller M, Putegnat J-B, Steyer J, Barrau S, Boissier F, et al. Inability of diaphragm ultrasound to predict extubation failure. *Chest*. 2019 Jun;155(6):1131–9.

29. Haaksma ME, Smit JM, Heldeweg MLA, Nooitgedacht JS, Atmowihardjo LN, Jonkman AH, et al. Holistic Ultrasound to Predict Extubation Failure in Clinical Practice. *Respiratory care*. 2021;66(6), 994-1003.

30. Llamas-Álvarez AM, Tenza-Lozano EM, Latour-Pérez J. Diaphragm and lung ultrasound to predict weaning outcome. *Chest*. 2017 Dec;152(6):1140–50.

31. Houston JG, Angus RM, Cowan MD, McMillan NC, Thomson NC. Ultrasound assessment of normal hemidiaphragmatic movement: relation to inspiratory volume. *Thorax*. 1994 May 1;49(5):500–3.

32. Spadaro S, Grasso S, Mauri T, Dalla Corte F, Alvisi V, Ragazzi R, et al. Can diaphragmatic ultrasonography performed during the T-tube trial predict weaning failure? The role of diaphragmatic rapid shallow breathing index. *Crit Care*. 2016;20:305

8

Diaphragmatic Ultrasound after Thoracic and Abdominal Surgery

Luigi Vetrugno, Daniele Orso, Elena Bignami, and Gianmaria Cammarota

Introduction

The diaphragm is like an engine piston, monotonously rising and falling throughout life, never stopping. Indeed, only as a result of drug-induced paralysis during anaesthesia or locoregional block does this muscle cease to work. At the end of anaesthesia, the capacity of the diaphragm to generate a trans-diaphragmatic pressure (Pdi) sufficient for patient ventilation autonomy is usually restored. In the past, only specialized centres were equipped with the instrumentation and expertise to measure diaphragmatic force. Two key methods were used. The first involved a double-balloon probe to measure the transdiaphragmatic pressure (Pdi, cm/H_2O); for this approach, one balloon is inserted into the oesophagus and the other goes into the stomach. The second key technique measures the twitch pressure (Pet, tw) – the pressure generated at the outer tip of the endotracheal tube [1]. Both methodologies require cervical magnetic stimulation of the phrenic nerve to produce an inspiratory effort. Today, point-of-care ultrasound (POCUS) offers an easy approach to diaphragm evaluation. It is simple to use, performed at the bedside, and repeatable over time.

Diaphragm ultrasound was first validated by Wait and colleagues in 1989 [2]; however, it has only recently gained ground in the field of anaesthesia thanks to research showing that the incidence of mechanical weaning failure, postoperative pulmonary complications, and length of hospital stay are all associated with a loss of diaphragm function after surgery [3–5].

DOI: 10.1201/9781003128694-11

The aim of this chapter is to highlight the use of POCUS for the early evaluation of diaphragmatic force in some specific types of cardiac, thoracic, and abdominal surgery, as well as orthopaedic surgical procedures requiring interscalene nerve block.

Cardiac Surgery

Respiratory complications are frequent after cardiac surgery and can contribute to morbidity, mortality, and increased healthcare costs [6, 7]. They include diaphragm dysfunction, and epidemiological data report the incidence of diaphragmatic paralysis after open cardiac surgery ranging from 30% to 75% [8]; however, the diagnosis of diaphragm dysfunction after cardiac surgery is most likely under-recognized, thus the prevalence of this complication under estimated. Phrenic nerve damage and consequent diaphragm dysfunction may also arise after cardiac surgery due to [9–11]:

1. The use of ice for myocardial protection – since the phrenic nerves, after the cervical region, cross the thoracic cavity close to the pericardium. To protect against damage and diaphragm dysfunction, insulation pads should be used.
2. Direct surgical damage of the left phrenic nerve (the left side being more affected than the right) after ligation of its blood supply during internal mammary artery dissection.
3. High cytokine levels and mitochondrial oxidative stress during cardio-pulmonary bypass (CPB). A role of these processes in diaphragm dysfunction was highlighted only recently. The high production of free radicals and reactive oxygen species during cardiac surgery leads to the activation of inflammatory and apoptotic pathways.

Diaphragmatic dysfunction is more frequently unilateral than bilateral. It must also be borne in mind that the left hemidiaphragm is more challenging to assess than the right hemidiaphragm [12]. Using new software and an anatomical motional (M)-mode for the ultrasound evaluation of diaphragmatic excursion, Pasero et al. were able to identify a greater proportion of patients exhibiting left diaphragm dysfunction following cardiac surgery [13]. The software used permits the free rotation to the M-mode line even if the acoustic window is not favourable for the good alignment of the ultrasound beam for left hemidiaphragmatic movements. An alternative solution, in the case of drainages and dressings inhibiting an anterior approach, would be the lateral approach as described by Lerolle et al. [14]. These authors found a linear correlation between excursion evaluated by ultrasound and the trans-diaphragmatic pressure gradient – an expression of the contribution of the diaphragm to the maximal inspiratory effort. Furthermore, Pierre-Henri Moury et al. recently assessed weaning from mechanical ventilation in cardiac surgical patients by evaluating diaphragm thickening during the spontaneous breathing trial (SBT) at the zone of apposition [15]. The authors found that diaphragm thickening could be markedly reduced in postoperative cardiac surgery, with 75% of patients found to have a thickening fraction (TF) less than 20%. This incidence was higher compared with those published by previous studies (reporting incidences around 60%). Diaphragmatic dysfunction in the study by Pierre-Henri Moury and colleagues mainly implied difficulty in weaning from invasive mechanical ventilation in the immediate postoperative period, and the authors did not correlate their data with respect to mechanical ventilation weaning failure.

Conversely, Bruni et al. showed that a diaphragm thickening fraction less than 20% was associated with a higher rate of difficult weaning, a lower 24-hour extubation rate, and a longer ICU length of stay [16]. Furthermore, in their study, a longer duration of surgery was associated with a greater reduction in diaphragm thickening. Moury et al. showed that diaphragm dysfunction resulted in an increase in hospital stay by 1 more day; moreover, three patients in this subgroup experienced extubation failure [15]. In the case of weaning difficulty, a higher exposure to the risks induced by invasive ventilation, such as the onset of nosocomial infections, particularly ventilator-associated pneumonia (VAP), increases the length of stay and the in-hospital mortality rate. Finally, POCUS diaphragm evaluation could provide a means for the early detection of diaphragm dysfunction, enabling strategies to be put into place (e.g., early physiotherapy) to mitigate the high risk of subsequent complications, such as pneumonia, sudden respiratory arrest, and prolonged mechanical ventilation complications [12, 17].

Thoracic Surgery

Depending on the intervention type, thoracotomy surgery is associated with postoperative pulmonary complications in 25–35% of patients, the occurrence of which may increase the probability of ICU admission, hospital length of stay, and mortality [18]. Direct injury to the diaphragm fibres or phrenic nerve and diaphragmatic weakness due to decreased postoperative mechanics play a significant role in the pathogenesis of pulmonary complications. However, their incidence seems to be lower after video-assisted thoracoscopic surgery (VATS) [19]. Recently, in an elegant work by Spadaro et al., which assessed postoperative patients in spontaneous breathing by means of the Boussuges technique, diaphragmatic dysfunction of less than 10 mm was found to positively correlate with the onset of post-surgical pulmonary complications [19]. Once again, their incidence was lower following VATS. Diaphragm dysfunction was diagnosed in 55% of patients undergoing video-assisted thoracoscopic surgery and in 83% in the thoracotomy group. A higher impairment in forced vital capacity was found in the latter. In this study, patients exhibiting diaphragmatic dysfunction within 24 hours after surgery also experienced more postoperative pulmonary complications. In the majority of cases, the ipsilateral diaphragm was involved.

As explained above, interventions within the upper thoracic region (for example, thymoma surgery) can cause damage to the phrenic nerve, and thus lead to diaphragm dysfunction. Cases of thymoma are frequently associated with neuromuscular disorders, such as myasthenia gravis, which may also involve the diaphragm [20]. Similarly, the use of muscle relaxants or corticosteroids in the case of a patient with some form of muscular asthenia can precipitate a borderline condition of compensated diaphragmatic dysfunction [21]. LoMauro et al. found diaphragm dysfunction to be common following bi-pulmonary transplant surgery, even in clinically silent forms or with subclinical manifestations [22].

In thoracic surgery, POCUS is proven to be a sufficiently reliable tool for establishing the presence and degree of postoperative diaphragmatic dysfunction. Diaphragmatic excursion and the thickening fraction correlate linearly with the forced vital capacity [19].

Upper Abdominal Surgery

POCUS is a practical modality for evaluating diaphragmatic function in patients after abdominal surgery. In the context of open major hepatic surgery and liver transplantation, right diaphragmatic dysfunction often occurs in the immediate postoperative period. McAllister and colleagues found that 79% of liver recipients suffered right phrenic nerve injury, and approximately half of these patients also exhibited hemidiaphragm paralysis [23]. Patients with unilateral diaphragmatic paralysis may often be asymptomatic in the immediate postoperative period. Diaphragm function recovers within a few months after surgery. Normal hemidiaphragm work can maintain adequate ventilation and gas exchange, both at rest and during mild exercise, through compensatory mechanisms in these patients.

The first case report to evidence the usefulness of POCUS following abdominal surgery for detecting diaphragmatic dysfunction as a cause of acute respiratory failure, with a resulting change in patient management, was presented by Barbariol and colleagues in 2015 [24].

Diaphragm ultrasound after abdominal surgery provides practical, functional information about the diaphragm and can also be easily repeated if follow-up is required. Some mechanisms of diaphragm dysfunction only come into play once abdominal surgery is concluded. For example, the long hours of traction exerted on the ribs by retractors during surgery can result in trauma to the muscle and phrenic nerves, damage which only becomes evident after surgery [25].

Retractors play a clear role in creating an adequately wide surgical field during an operation. The retractor is usually secured to the patient's bed by means of the upright metal bar. The valves applied to the wound are moved by metal cables retracted by a pulley placed on the metal arch, and a sliding cable fixes the retraction in the desired position. In this way, the upper abdomen and the patient's organs are optimally exposed.

The pulmonary bases on the right are reduced following upper abdominal surgery with traction, and the consequent diaphragm dysfunction plays a central role in determining atelectasis. According to retrospective data, pulmonary complications occur in around 20% of patients under these circumstances [25]. Kim et al., in 35 patients undergoing hepatic lobectomy, demonstrated that the use of ultrasound evaluation in M-mode could help monitor diaphragmatic recovery [26]. The inspiratory diaphragmatic amplitude was shown to linearly correlate with vital capacity (sensitivity from 80% to 94% and specificity from 76% to 91%, depending on the cut-off used). Pain is the second most important factor, with the abdominal wound discouraging patients from employing their full respiratory range, who instead activate the diaphragm to produce shorter and more shallow breaths. Since surgical dressings also limit the muscular motion of a patient's abdomen, this lack of freedom of movement also affects the diaphragm.

The issue of intra-abdominal hypertension (IAH), defined as an abdominal pressure that exceeds 12 mmHg in at least three consecutive assessments performed within a time window of 4–6 h, must also be mentioned here. Abdominal hypertension can transform into abdominal compartment syndrome (ACS) if the intra-abdominal pressure (IAP) exceeds 20 mmHg, with associated single or multiple organ dysfunction/failure [27]. The prevalence of IAH varies in the literature according to the different patient populations, reaching 65% in surgical ICU patients and 32% in combined medical–surgical patients. The primary mechanical effects through which IAH affects respiratory function are a decreased compliance of the thoracic–pulmonary system and an upward displacement of the diaphragm; the consequent atelectasis may trigger pneumonia. In this case, diaphragm movement is reduced or absent [27, 28].

A Concept in Development

Since Stephen Hales's first observations on the diaphragm's functioning kinetics in the early 18th century, this organ's role on the hemodynamics of the systemic circulation and the thoracic and abdominal organs has been clear [29, 30]. The pressure gradient created by the movement variation promotes the flow of venous blood to the heart from the liver, and from the abdominal compartment to the inferior vena cava. Rabinovici and colleagues were among the first to observe in animal models an alternating fluctuation of the caval flow during the respiratory cycle [31].

Other studies have confirmed the diaphragm's impact on venous return and highlighted the effects on portal return. An adequate blood supply to the liver, with a difference in pressure between the portal vein and the hepatic veins and the inferior vena cava, is essential for good liver function. Therefore, it is important to estimate the share/distribution of venous return between the vena cava and portal flow depending on the diaphragmatic movement during the breathing cycle. Furthermore, Tain-Yen Hsia et al. more recently showed how respiration has important influences on venous return in patients with Fontan's anomaly, and the increase in the amount coming from the transhepatic portal circulation [32]. Thus, diaphragm function plays a central role in the dynamics of thoracic and abdominal blood flows, with an important effect on hepatic inflow and outflow. However, this aspect has yet to be fully understood.

Shoulder Surgery (Diaphragmatic Paralysis after Interscalene Block)

Over recent years, locoregional anaesthetic techniques have become increasingly popular for use in orthopaedic surgery: shoulder, clavicle, and superior limb surgery in particular. The benefits of locoregional anaesthesia include a lower incidence of pulmonary complications, fewer ICU admissions, and faster recovery. However, locoregional blocks present important risks that must be recognized and taken into consideration. Cervical plexus nerve block, and interscalenic nerve block (INB) in particular, are more susceptible to accidental phrenic nerve paralysis due to the anatomical arrangement of these nerve trunks [33, 34]. For example, after INB and the supraclavicular block, hemidiaphragm paresis has been reported in up to 92% and 65% of cases, respectively [35].

Pakala et al. reported a series of nine cases of hemidiaphragm dysfunction after INB, with an incidence rate of approximately one per 2,000 patients [33]. However, this rate probably only reflects the incidence of dysfunction with clinical manifestations. Considering that 55% of patients with diaphragm dysfunction are asymptomatic [33], the above reported incidence of hemidiaphragm paralysis associated with INB is certainly underestimated. Therefore, more research into this collateral effect in patients with chronic obstructive pulmonary disease, obesity, sleep apnea syndrome, or chest trauma before surgery is required.

Nevertheless, INB remains one of the most widely used anaesthetic and analgesic techniques for shoulder surgery. Recent studies have investigated phrenic-sparing alternative approaches to analgesia. Renes et al. demonstrated that an ultrasound-guided posterior-lateral supraclavicular block using 20 mL of local anaesthetic resulted in no cases of hemidiaphragm paralysis in a sample of 30 patients [36]. Thus, thanks to their more distal position away from the phrenic nerve, supraclavicular brachial plexus blocks

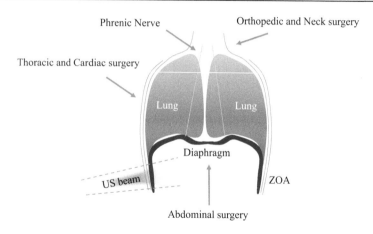

Figure 8.1 Potential surgical insult on the diaphragm

are recommended to reduce the incidence of hemidiaphragmatic paralysis. In this clinical context, a recently published case study illustrated the use of a refined ultrasound-guided variation of the interscalene block: the superior trunk block. The superior trunk block was performed on a pulmonary-compromised patient using a small volume of anaesthesia (12 mL); POCUS confirmed the lack of any consequent hemidiaphragmatic paralysis [36]. That said, a locoregional anaesthesia technique for shoulder surgery devoid of any risk of hemidiaphragmatic paralysis has yet to be demonstrated. So, bearing in mind that diaphragm dysfunction following nerve block takes some time to recover, and, in the worst cases, may even constitute permanent nerve damage, it is advisable to check diaphragm function both before performing an INB block and after recovery.

Regarding the best acoustic approaches to the diaphragm, the liver provides a very good window for the measurement of diaphragm excursion on the right side, whereas the window on the left side via the spleen is difficult due to the presence of the stomach and its contents. If a left side approach is required, we suggest the lateral one, as proposed by Lerolle et al. [14].

Finally, it should be remembered that, similar to some other types of surgery (namely, carotid surgery), an equivalent anesthetic efficacy can be obtained for clavicle surgery using superficial cervical plexus block alone or in association with INB for postoperative pain. Thus, the possibility of using the first block only can minimize the risk of damage to the phrenic nerve [37].

Conclusion

The evaluation of diaphragm excursion using ultrasound is an easy skill to master, with just 25 supervised procedures necessary to become proficient. On the other hand, evaluation of the diaphragm thickening fraction is more complicated, requiring more expert operators. With this in mind, the introduction of diaphragmatic ultrasound before and after cardiac, thoracic, abdominal, and orthopedic surgery should be considered for its potential to provide meaningful information pertinent to pathophysiological processes afflicting the diaphragm, which can in turn lead to improvements in patient outcome.

References

1. Dres M, Goligher EC, Heunks LMA, Brochard LJ. Critical illness-associated diaphragm weakness. *Intensive Care Med.* 2017 Oct;43(10):1441–1452. doi: 10.1007/s00134-017-4928-4. Epub 2017 Sep 15. PMID: 28917004.

2. Wait JL, Nahormek PA, Yost WT, Rochester DP. Diaphragmatic thickness-lung volume relationship in vivo. *J Appl Physiol* (1985). 1989 Oct;67(4):1560–8. doi: 10.1152/jappl.1989.67.4.1560. PMID: 2676955.

3. Goligher EC, Brochard LJ, Reid WD, Fan E, Saarela O, Slutsky AS, Kavanagh BP, Rubenfeld GD, Ferguson ND. Diaphragmatic myotrauma: a mediator of prolonged ventilation and poor patient outcomes in acute respiratory failure. *Lancet Respir Med.* 2019 Jan;7(1):90–98. doi: 10.1016/S2213-2600(18)30366-7. Epub 2018 Nov 16. PMID: 30455078.

4. Demoule A, Jung B, Prodanovic H, Molinari N, Chanques G, Coirault C, Matecki S, Duguet A, Similowski T, Jaber S. Diaphragm dysfunction on admission to the intensive care unit. Prevalence, risk factors, and prognostic impact-a prospective study. *Am J Respir Crit Care Med.* 2013 Jul 15;188(2):213–9. doi: 10.1164/rccm.201209-1668OC. PMID: 23641946.

5. Moury PH, Cuisinier A, Durand M, Bosson JL, Chavanon O, Payen JF, Jaber S, Albaladejo P. Diaphragm thickening in cardiac surgery: a perioperative prospective ultrasound study. *Ann Intensive Care.* 2019 Apr 24;9(1):50. doi: 10.1186/s13613-019-0521-z. PMID: 31016412; PMCID: PMC6478777.

6. Branca P, McGaw P, Light R. Factors associated with prolonged mechanical ventilation following coronary artery bypass surgery. *Chest.* 2001 Feb;119(2):537–46. doi: 10.1378/chest.119.2.537. PMID: 11171735.

7. García-Delgado M, Navarrete-Sánchez I, Colmenero M. Preventing and managing perioperative pulmonary complications following cardiac surgery. *Curr Opin Anaesthesiol.* 2014 Apr;27(2):146–52. doi: 10.1097/ACO.0000000000000059. PMID: 24514031.

8. Mehta Y, Vats M, Singh A, Trehan N. Incidence and management of diaphragmatic palsy in patients after cardiac surgery. *Indian J Crit Care Med.* 2008 Jul;12(3):91–5. doi: 10.4103/0972-5229.43676. PMID: 19742255; PMCID: PMC2738314.

9. Aguirre VJ, Sinha P, Zimmet A, Lee GA, Kwa L, Rosenfeldt F. Phrenic nerve injury during cardiac surgery: mechanisms, management and prevention. *Heart Lung Circ.* 2013 Nov;22(11):895–902. doi: 10.1016/j.hlc.2013.06.010. Epub 2013 Aug 13. PMID: 23948287.

10. Bignami E, Guarnieri M, Saglietti F, Ramelli A, Vetrugno L. Diaphragmatic dysfunction following cardiac surgery: is there a role for pulmonary ultrasound? *J Cardiothorac Vasc Anesth.* 2018 Oct;32(5):e6–e7. doi: 10.1053/j.jvca.2018.04.054. Epub 2018 May 1. PMID: 29804687.

11. Jellish WS, Oftadeh M. Peripheral nerve injury in cardiac surgery. *J Cardiothorac Vasc Anesth.* 2018 Feb;32(1):495–511. doi: 10.1053/j.jvca.2017.08.030. Epub 2017 Aug 19. PMID: 29248326.

12. Vetrugno L, Guadagnin GM, Barbariol F, Langiano N, Zangrillo A, Bove T. Ultrasound imaging for diaphragm dysfunction: a narrative literature review. *J Cardiothorac Vasc Anesth*. 2019 Sep;33(9):2525–2536. doi: 10.1053/j.jvca.2019.01.003. Epub 2019 Jan 4. PMID: 30686657.

13. Pasero D, Koeltz A, Placido R, Fontes Lima M, Haun O, Rienzo M, Marrache D, Pirracchio R, Safran D, Cholley B. Improving ultrasonic measurement of diaphragmatic excursion after cardiac surgery using the anatomical M-mode: a randomized crossover study. *Intensive Care Med*. 2015 Apr;41(4):650–6. doi: 10.1007/s00134-014-3625-9. Epub 2015 Jan 9. PMID: 25573500.

14. Lerolle N, Guérot E, Dimassi S, Zegdi R, Faisy C, Fagon JY, Diehl JL. Ultrasonographic diagnostic criterion for severe diaphragmatic dysfunction after cardiac surgery. *Chest*. 2009 Feb;135(2):401–407. doi: 10.1378/chest.08-1531. Epub 2008 Aug 27. PMID: 18753469.

15. Moury PH, Cuisinier A, Durand M, Bosson JL, Chavanon O, Payen JF, Jaber S, Albaladejo P. Diaphragm thickening in cardiac surgery: a perioperative prospective ultrasound study. *Ann Intensive Care*. 2019 Apr 24;9(1):50. doi: 10.1186/s13613-019-0521-z. PMID: 31016412; PMCID: PMC6478777.

16. Bruni A, Garofalo E, Pasin L, Serraino GF, Cammarota G, Longhini F, Landoni G, Lembo R, Mastroroberto P, Navalesi P, MaGIC (Magna Graecia Intensive care and Cardiac surgery) Group. Diaphragmatic dysfunction after elective cardiac surgery: a prospective observational study. *J Cardiothorac Vasc Anesth*. 2020 Dec;34(12):3336–3344. doi: 10.1053/j.jvca.2020.06.038. Epub 2020 Jun 17. PMID: 32653270.

17. Dres M, Demoule A. Diaphragm dysfunction during weaning from mechanical ventilation: an underestimated phenomenon with clinical implications. Crit Care. 2018 Mar 20;22(1):73. doi: 10.1186/s13054-018-1992-2. PMID: 29558983; PMCID: PMC5861656.

18. Miskovic A, Lumb AB. Postoperative pulmonary complications. *Br J Anaesth*. 2017 Mar 1;118(3):317–334. doi: 10.1093/bja/aex002. PMID: 28186222.

19. Spadaro S, Grasso S, Dres M, Fogagnolo A, Dalla Corte F, Tamburini N, Maniscalco P, Cavallesco G, Alvisi V, Stripoli T, De Camillis E, Ragazzi R, Volta CA. Point of care ultrasound to identify diaphragmatic dysfunction after thoracic surgery. *Anesthesiology*. 2019 Aug;131(2):266–278. doi: 10.1097/ALN.0000000000002774. PMID: 31166236.

20. McCaul JA, Hislop WS. Transient hemi-diaphragmatic paralysis following neck surgery: report of a case and review of the literature. *J R Coll Surg Edinb*. 2001 Jun;46(3):186–8. PMID: 11478021.

21. Quint LE. Thoracic complications and emergencies in oncologic patients. *Cancer Imaging*. 2009 Oct 2;9 Spec No A(Special issue A):S75–82. doi: 10.1102/1470-7330.2009.9031. PMID: 19965299; PMCID: PMC2797469.

22. LoMauro A, Righi I, Privitera E, Vergari M, Nigro M, Aliverti A, Frykholm P, Tarsia P, Morlacchi L, Nosotti M, Palleschi A. The impaired diaphragmatic function after bilateral lung transplantation: A multifactorial longitudinal study. *J Heart Lung Transplant*. 2020 Aug;39(8):795–804. doi: 10.1016/j.healun.2020.04.010. Epub 2020 Apr 21. PMID: 32362476.

23. McAlister VC, Grant DR, Roy A, Brown WF, Hutton LC, Leasa DJ, Ghent CN, Veitch JE, Wall WJ. Right phrenic nerve injury in orthotopic liver transplantation. *Transplantation*. 1993 Apr;55(4):826–30. doi: 10.1097/00007890-199304000-00027. PMID: 8475559.

24. Barbariol F, Vetrugno L, Pompei L, De Flaviis A, Rocca GD. Point-of-care ultrasound of the diaphragm in a liver transplant patient with acute respiratory failure. *Crit Ultrasound J*. 2015 Mar 28;7:3. doi: 10.1186/s13089-015-0021-9. PMID: 25859317; PMCID: PMC4388066.

25. Fayssoil A, Behin A, Ogna A, Mompoint D, Amthor H, Clair B, Laforet P, Mansart A, Prigent H, Orlikowski D, Stojkovic T, Vinit S, Carlier R, Eymard B, Lofaso F, Annane D. Diaphragm: pathophysiology and ultrasound imaging in neuromuscular disorders. *J Neuromuscul Dis*. 2018;5(1):1–10. doi: 10.3233/JND-170276. PMID: 29278898; PMCID: PMC5836400.

26. Kim SH, Na S, Choi JS, Na SH, Shin S, Koh SO. An evaluation of diaphragmatic movement by M-mode sonography as a predictor of pulmonary dysfunction after upper abdominal surgery. *Anesth Analg*. 2010 May 1;110(5):1349–54. doi: 10.1213/ANE.0b013e3181d5e4d8. PMID: 20418298.

27. Vetrugno L, Brussa A, Guadagnin GM, Orso D, De Lorenzo F, Cammarota G, Santangelo E, Bove T. Mechanical ventilation weaning issues can be counted on the fingers of just one hand: part 2. *Ultrasound J*. 2020 Mar 13;12(1):15. doi: 10.1186/s13089-020-00160-z. PMID: 32166639; PMCID: PMC7067962.

28. Vetrugno L, Guadagnin GM, Brussa A, Orso D, Garofalo E, Bruni A, Longhini F, Bove T. Mechanical ventilation weaning issues can be counted on the fingers of just one hand: part 1. *Ultrasound J*. 2020 Mar 13;12(1):9. doi: 10.1186/s13089-020-00161-y. PMID: 32166566; PMCID: PMC7067937.

29. West JB. Stephen Hales: neglected respiratory physiologist. *J Appl Physiol Respir Environ Exerc Physiol*. 1984 Sep;57(3):635–9. doi: 10.1152/jappl.1984.57.3.635. PMID: 6386767.

30. Eknoyan, G. Stephen Hales: the contributions of an Enlightenment physiologist to the study of the kidney in health and disease. *G Ital Nefrol*. 2016 Feb;33(Suppl 66):33.S66.5. PMID: 26913873.

31. Rabinovici N, Navot N. The relationship between respiration, pressure and flow distribution in the vena cava and portal and hepatic veins. *Surg Gynecol Obstet*. 1980 Dec;151(6):753–63. PMID: 7444726.

32. Hsia TY, Khambadkone S, Redington AN, Migliavacca F, Deanfield JE, de Leval MR. Effects of respiration and gravity on infradiaphragmatic venous flow in normal and Fontan patients. *Circulation*. 2000 Nov 7;102(19 Suppl 3):III148–53. doi: 10.1161/01.cir.102.suppl_3.iii-148. PMID: 11082378.

33. Pakala SR, Beckman JD, Lyman S, Zayas VM. Cervical spine disease is a risk factor for persistent phrenic nerve paresis following interscalene nerve block. *Reg Anesth Pain Med*. 2013 May-Jun;38(3):239–42. doi: 10.1097/AAP.0b013e318289e922. PMID: 23518866.

34. Khurana J, Gartner SC, Naik L, Tsui BCH. Ultrasound identification of diaphragm by novices using ABCDE technique. *Reg Anesth Pain Med*. 2018 Feb;43(2):161–165. doi: 10.1097/AAP.0000000000000718. PMID: 29315130.

35. El-Boghdadly K, Chin KJ, Chan VWS. Phrenic nerve palsy and regional anesthesia for shoulder surgery: anatomical, physiologic, and clinical considerations. *Anesthesiology.* 2017 Jul;127(1):173–191. doi: 10.1097/ALN.0000000000001668. PMID: 28514241.

36. Renes SH, Spoormans HH, Gielen MJ, Rettig HC, van Geffen GJ. Hemidiaphragmatic paresis can be avoided in ultrasound-guided supraclavicular brachial plexus block. *Reg Anesth Pain Med.* 2009 Nov-Dec;34(6):595–9. doi: 10.1097/aap.0b013e3181bfbd83. PMID: 19916254.

37. Divella M, Vetrugno L. Regional blocks for clavicle fractures: keep Hippocrates in mind. *Minerva Anestesiol.* 2021 Mar 10. doi: 10.23736/S0375-9393.21.15630-5. Epub ahead of print. PMID: 33688703.

9

Diaphragm Ultrasound in Patients with Neuromuscular Disorders

Abdallah Fayssoil

Introduction

Neuromuscular disorders are a group of neurological diseases that can affect the muscles, the neuromuscular junction, the peripheral nerves, and the motor neurons. Respiratory function can be affected progressively in muscular respiratory. The diaphragm is particularly affected in late onset Pompe disease (LOPD). Clinical symptoms of NMD patients with diaphragm dysfunction can be subtle particularly in patients with peripheral skeletal disabilities. Patients may disclose dyspnea, morning headache, fatigue, nocturnal awakenings, and hypersomnia (1). Abnormal sleep disorders are frequent in NMD patients with diaphragm dysfunction (2). Diurnal hypoventilation may occur later with disease progression. Even if the introduction of non-invasive ventilation has improved survival in muscular dystrophy (3, 4), NMD exposes patients to a risk of acute respiratory failure (5). The diaphragm is the main inspiratory muscle that accounts for more than 80% of forced vital capacity in healthy persons. An ultrasound is a non-invasive radiological technique that can be used to assess diaphragm morphology and function in neuromuscular disorders. A diaphragm ultrasound can be performed in outclinic patients but also in patients admitted in hospital because of acute respiratory distress.

Pathophysiology of Respiration Function in Neuromuscular Disorders

In patients with neuromuscular diseases, the onset of weakness of the inspiratory muscles and weakness of the expiratory muscles leads progressively to a reduction of lung volumes (pulmonary vital capacity, total lung capacity, functional residual capacity). In addition, chest wall compliance decreases in relation to stiffening of thorax and scoliosis, particularly

DOI: 10.1201/9781003128694-12

in patients with Duchenne muscular dystrophy. Furthermore, lung compliance decreases, due to microatelectasia and recurrent aspirations (6). The upper airway is also affected in NMD and the presence of hypotonia may increase upper airway resistance that contributes to the increase of the respiratory workload (7). In response to respiratory muscle weakness, the respiratory drive increases. However, hypoventilation occurs when the compensatory mechanism becomes insufficient to cope with the increase of the respiratory load (8). Finally, cough function is altered and the eventual presence of swallowing derangement increases the risk of aspiration and the risk of acute respiratory failure (6).

In clinic, patients with diaphragm dysfunction may disclose a paradoxical inward motion where the ribcage is expanding. This phenomenon occurs particularly in the supine position. In fact, in normal situations, the contraction of the diaphragm generates a decrease of pleural pressure, an increase of the abdominal pressure leading to an outward displacement of the abdominal wall and a displacement of the lower rib cage, in relation to the appositional force (9).

Diaphragm Ultrasound

Traditional techniques used to assess the diaphragm include measurement of maximal inspiratory pressure (MIP), delta forced vital capacity (VC), sniff nasal inspiratory pressure, and the transdiaphragmatic pressures that remain the gold standard to assess diaphragm strength. A decline in FVC of more than 20% from sitting position to supine position is a hallmark of diaphragm weakness (10). MIP provides a global assessment of the inspiratory muscles that include the diaphragm and the accessory inspiratory muscles whereas diaphragm ultrasound focuses on the diaphragm evaluation. In addition, transdiaphragmatic measurement requires an invasive approach that cannot be performed routinely in patients with neuromuscular disorders.

Ultrasound emerged as a non-invasive technic to assess and follow patients with neuromuscular disorders. Ultrasound can provide an assessment of diaphragm thickness and diaphragm motion with higher reproducibility (11, 12) and this technique can be performed at bedside. Ultrasound may help to search for early respiratory involvement in patients with NMD. Diaphragm ultrasound parameters are significantly associated with inspiratory muscles strength and lung function in health persons (13) and in patients with neuromuscular disorders (14, 15). The diaphragm can be analyzed using ultrasound at rest breathing, deep breathing, and during sniff manoeuvre.

Diaphragm thickness is measured at the apposition zone, using a transducer placed perpendicularly to the chest wall, between the antero-axillary line and the mid-axillary line (Figure 9.1). For this measurement, it is usual to use a linear probe with higher frequency. With B mode, the diaphragm was visualized as a hypoechogenic layer of muscle tissue surrounded by two hyperechogenic lines, namely the pleural line and the peritoneal line. Diaphragm thickness was measured at end of the expiratory phase and at the end of a deep inspiration. Diaphragm thickening was defined as percentage ratio between end inspiratory thickness and end expiratory thickness, as described in Chapter 4 (16). To assess the diaphragm motion, a cardiac probe is used. It is placed in the anterior subcostal region, providing the subcostal view, using M mode. From this view, the diaphragm motion can be measured at rest, during deep inspiration or during a sniff manoeuvre, with M mode (16). The right diaphragm is assessed through the liver window and the left diaphragm through the spleen window.

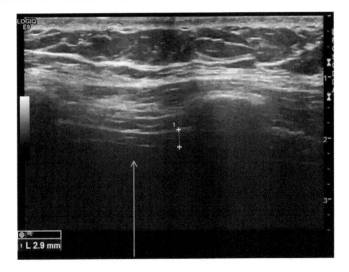

Figure 9.1 Right diaphragm thickness measurement (arrow) in a patient with myotonic dystrophy type 1 using ultrasound

Diaphragm Ultrasound in Neuromuscular Disorders in a Neuromuscular Centre

Patients with NMD are followed classically in outclinic in a multidisciplinary team that involves cardiologists, pneumologists, neurologists, psychologists, and physiotherapists. Diaphragm ultrasound can be performed in the context of outclinic but also in the context of an acute respiratory failure, unexplained weaning failure, and myasthenia crisis.

Neuromuscular disorders encompass a wide spectrum of diseases ranging from muscular dystrophies to diseases that affect the motor neurons (Table 9.1).

ALS is a degenerative neuromuscular disorder with a worse prognosis. The disease affects upper motor neurons and lower motor neurons. Clinical findings include pseudo bulbar derangement, hyperreflexia, and spasticity. Physical examination may find muscle atrophy, weakness, and fasciculations. Diagnosis relies on clinic and electromyography (17). Respiratory insufficiency occurs during the course of the disease and is the main cause of death. Monitoring respiratory function is essential in this disease. Tests used to follow ALS patients include measurements of forced VC, Motor Unit Number Estimation (MUNE), and ALS Functional Rating Scale (ALSFRS) (18). Diaphragm function is affected in ALS and diaphragm US can be used to monitor patients with ALS (17). In ALS, diaphragm thickness at rest and at inspiration are reduced compared to healthy persons (19). Yoshioka et al. (20) reported cases series of clinical application of ultrasound to evaluate diaphragm weakness, diaphragm paralysis and diaphragm atrophy in ALS (20). In fact, a significant association between the diaphragm end inspiratory thickness measured with US and the peak-to-peak amplitude of the diaphragmatic motor response to phrenic nerve stimulation in patients with ALS (21). Hiwatani et al. (22) reported a significant association between VC and diaphragm end inspiratory thickness, diaphragm end expiratory thickness and diaphragm thickening ratio. Diaphragm ultrasound parameters were reduced in ALS patients with a pulmonary VC < 80% (22). Sartucci et al. (19) found in ALS patients a significant correlation between

Table 9.1 Neuromuscular disorders with respiratory involvement

Myopathy	Neuromuscular junction	Motor nerves
• LOPD • Steinert disease Duchenne muscular dystrophy • Becker muscular dystrophy • Sarcoglycanopathy • Calpainothies • Congenital myopathy • FSHD1 • Collagen VI myopathies • Myositis	• Myasthenia gravis • Toxics • Botulism	• ALS • SMA • Guillian Barre syndrome • Toxics • Critical illness neuropathy

diaphragm ultrasound and respiratory function parameters (forced VC and FEV) as well as a significant correlation between diaphragm ultrasound and clinical scores. In conclusion, ALS, diaphragm ultrasound can be used to assess patients with dyspnea, screen patients at risk of respiratory insufficiency, and monitor patients (17).

Spinal muscular atrophies (SMA) are neuromuscular disorders in relation to defect in the survival motor neuron (SMN1) gene. The disease is characterized by a progressive degeneration of spinal cord motor neurons and patients disclose weakness and atrophy of skeletal muscles (23). The most severe form is the type 1 SMA that is characterized by weakness, severe hypotonia, swallowing disorders and respiratory failure over the first year of life (24). Ultrasound can be used to assess patients in this disease particularly, SMA patients with acute respiratory distress (25).

LOPD is an autosomal recessive lysosomal storage disease in relation to deficiency in alpha 1,4 glucosidase enzyme. Clinical pattern includes progressive limb-girdle muscle weakness associated with diaphragm weakness (15). In the study by Ruggeri et al. (15), that included patients with LOPD, diaphragm thickness at FRC was significantly associated with MIP (r 0.74 p < 0.0001) and forced VC (r 0.73 p < 0.05). Diaphragm thickening fraction was significantly associated win inspiratory muscles strength (r 0.80 p < 0.001 between TF and MIP) and forced VC (r 0.66 p < 0.005) (15).

Diaphragm inspiratory motion is also significantly associated with lung volumes and inspiratory muscles strength (r 0.79 p < 0.005 between diaphragm inspiratory motion and FVC and r 0.81 p < 0.005 between diaphragm inspiratory motion and MIP) (15). Another study (26) reported similar findings with a reduction of forced VC and MIP in LOPD; these previous parameters were significantly correlated with clinical disease severity in LOPD (r 0.72 between FVC and Walton and Gardner-Medwin scale) (26). Sniff manoeuvre can be coupled with ultrasound to assess diaphragm in LOPD, since sniff diaphragm peak velocity are reduced in LOPD (26). Finally, sniff TM mode can be used to search for diaphragm weakness or paralysis in LOPD, searching for paradoxical diaphragm motion (27).

Collagen VI myopathy is another hereditary myopathy that can affect diaphragm function (28). Collagen VI myopathy is in relation to mutations in the COL6A1-3 genes. These diseases include Ullrich congenital muscular dystrophy, the most severe form, and Bethlem myopathy, the milder form (28).

Myotonic dystrophy type 1 (DM1) is a frequent neuromuscular disorder with a hereditary autosomal dominant pattern, caused by an unstable cytosine-thymine-guanine (CTG) repeat expansion in the 3' untranslated region (3'UTR) of the dystrophia myotonica protein kinase (DMPK) gene (29). Clinical features include cardiac arrhythmia, cardiac conduction defects, respiratory insufficiency, endocrine system, and ophthalmologic impairment. Life expectancy is reduced in DM1 with a mean age of death around 54 years, as the consequence of respiratory failure in most than 50% of cases (5). Respiratory involvement is frequent in patients with DM1, consisting of a restrictive pattern, in relation to weakness of respiratory muscles (30). This respiratory feature is characterized by a progressive annual VC decline over time (31). In a recent study that included DM1 patients, Henke et al. (32) reported a reduced diaphragm thickening ratio (diaphragm thickness at TLC / diaphragm thickness at FRC) in DM1 patients, and this parameter is significantly correlated with muscular impairment rating (MIRS) score. Sniff diaphragm motion or tissue Doppler peak velocity sniff are significantly associated with sniff nasal pressure in DM 1 (14). These previous parameters can predict respiratory involvement in patients with myotonic muscular dystrophy (14).

Facioscapulohumeral muscular dystrophy (FSHD1) is one of the most common hereditary muscular dystrophy characterized by facial and shoulder weakness, in relation to a contraction of the subtelomeric D4Z4 repeat on chromosome 4q35. clinical presentation may vary with an asymmetric muscle involvement and respiratory muscles may be involved (33). A shorter D4Z4 repeat has been reported to be associated with earlier disease onset (34). Respiratory involvement is frequent in FSHD1 patients in wheelchairs and patients with severe clinical disease and proximal lower limbs weakness (35, 36). Ultrasound can be used for the evaluation of FSHD1 patients. Diaphragm inspiration motion and diaphragm thickening ratio are reduced in FSHD1 in comparison with healthy persons (37). MIP is significantly associated with diaphragm thickening ratio and with diaphragm inspiratory motion in FSHD1 (37). Ultrasound may reveal diaphragm asymmetric inspiratory pattern (38) (Figures 9.2a and 9.2b).

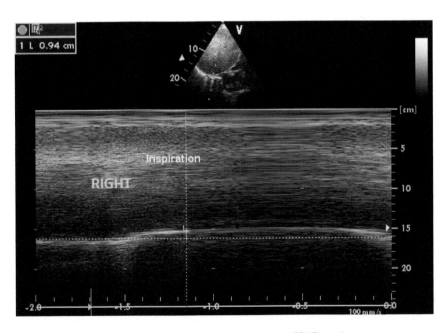

Figure 9.2a Reduced right diaphragmatic inspiratory motion in an FSHD1 patient

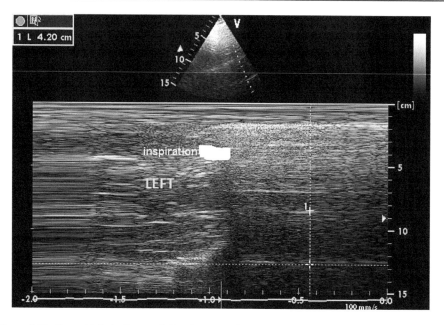

Figure 9.2b Correct left diaphragmatic inspiratory motion in the same FSHD1 patient. Note the asymmetric diaphragm motion between the right and the left hemidiaphragm

Duchenne muscular dystrophy (DMD) is a neuromuscular disease, due to dystrophin gene defect. This disease is characterized by a progressive reduction of lung volumes with the onset of a restrictive pulmonary pattern, nocturnal followed by diurnal hypoventilation (39). Ultrasound can be used in DMD to assess and follow the respiratory status. Diaphragm thickness is lower in DMD patients in comparison with healthy persons (40). In addition, diaphragm ultrasound parameters decrease with age in DMD (41). Finally, tissue Doppler imaging can be used to monitor diaphragm function (Figure 9.3).

Becker muscular dystrophy (BMD) is an X linked disease caused by mutations that affect DMD gene encoding the dystrophin protein (42). This disease is characterized by a milder phenotype and a milder course in comparison with Duchenne muscular dystrophy (DMD). Restrictive pulmonary pattern may be present in patients with BMD (42).

Myasthenia gravis (MG) is the most common disorder that affects the neuromuscular junction of skeletal muscles. This disease is often in relation to the presence of autoantibodies against acetylcholine receptors in the post synaptic area. Patients with MG are at risk of myasthenia crisis that is characterized by a worsening of muscle weakness, leading to acute respiratory failure (43). Myasthenic crisis may be in relation to the weakness of respiratory muscles and or weakness of upper airway muscles leading to obstruction and aspiration (44). This complication requires the introduction of mechanical ventilation. About one-fifth of MG patients will experience myasthenia crisis (44). Ultrasound can be used to evaluate the respiratory status of patients and may help to guide therapeutic in acute situations. A recent case report highlights the usefulness of diaphragm ultrasound to guide plasma exchange therapy in patients with myasthenia crisis (45).

Guillain-Barre syndrome is an acute inflammatory polyneuropathy that can affect the respiratory function. Risk factors for acute respiratory insufficiency include facial

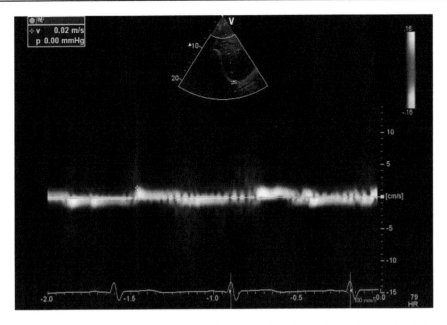

Figure 9.3 Diaphragm Tissue Doppler imaging. Note the significant reduction of the peak inspiratory velocity in a DMD patient with restrictive respiratory insufficiency

palsy, bulbar weakness, and low neck MRC (Medical Research Council) score (46, 47). It is important to stratify patients with this disease. Diaphragm ultrasound may help to search for early respiratory involvement in order to better provide respiratory assistance (46).

Conclusion

Diaphragm ultrasound is a single radiological technique that can be used at bedside to evaluate and monitor patients with neuromuscular disorders. This technique can be integrated into the multidisciplinary approach in the management of NMD patients. In acute and subacute situations, ultrasound can help to stratify patients and to screen patients at risk of acute respiratory failure that will require mechanical ventilation.

References

1. McCool FD, Tzelepis GE. Dysfunction of the diaphragm. *N Engl J Med.* 2012 Mar 8;366(10):932–42.
2. Ragette R, Mellies U, Schwake C, Voit T, Teschler H. Patterns and predictors of sleep disordered breathing in primary myopathies. *Thorax.* 2002 Aug;57(8):724–8.
3. Vivekananda U, Turner C. A model to predict ventilator requirement in myotonic dystrophy type 1. *Muscle Nerve.* 2019 Jun;59(6):683–7.

4. Nugent AM, Smith IE, Shneerson JM. Domiciliary-assisted ventilation in patients with myotonic dystrophy. *Chest*. 2002 Feb;121(2):459–64.

5. Mathieu J, Allard P, Potvin L, Prévost C, Bégin P. A 10-year study of mortality in a cohort of patients with myotonic dystrophy. *Neurology*. 1999 May 12;52(8):1658–62.

6. Benditt JO. Pathophysiology of neuromuscular respiratory diseases. *Clin Chest Med*. 2018 Jun;39(2):297–308.

7. Eikermann M, Vogt FM, Herbstreit F, Vahid-Dastgerdi M, Zenge MO, Ochterbeck C, de Greiff A, Peters J. The predisposition to inspiratory upper airway collapse during partial neuromuscular blockade. *Am J Respir Crit Care Med*. 2007 Jan 1;175(1):9–15.

8. Fauroux B, Khirani S. Neuromuscular disease and respiratory physiology in children: putting lung function into perspective. *Respirology*. 2014 Aug;19(6):782–91.

9. Green M, Moxham J. The respiratory muscles. *Clin Sci*. 1985;68(1):1–10.

10. Perrin C, Unterborn JN, Ambrosio CD, Hill NS. Pulmonary complications of chronic neuromuscular diseases and their management. *Muscle Nerve*. 2004 Jan;29(1):5–27.

11. Scarlata S, Mancini D, Laudisio A, Raffaele AI. Reproducibility of diaphragmatic thickness measured by M-mode ultrasonography in healthy volunteers. *Respir Physiol Neurobiol*. 2019 Feb;260:58–62.

12. Boussuges A, Gole Y, Blanc P. Diaphragmatic motion studied by m-mode ultrasonography: methods, reproducibility, and normal values. *Chest*. 2009 Feb;135(2):391–400.

13. Cardenas LZ, Santana PV, Caruso P, Ribeiro de Carvalho CR, Pereira de Albuquerque AL. Diaphragmatic ultrasound correlates with inspiratory muscle strength and pulmonary function in healthy subjects. *Ultrasound Med Biol*. 2018 Apr;44(4):786–793.

14. Fayssoil A, Nguyen LS, Ogna A, Stojkovic T, Meng P, Mompoint D, Carlier R, Prigent H, Clair B, Behin A, Laforet P, Bassez G, Crenn P, Orlikowski D, Annane D, Eymard B, Lofaso F. Diaphragm sniff ultrasound: Normal values, relationship with sniff nasal pressure and accuracy for predicting respiratory involvement in patients with neuromuscular disorders. *PLoS One*. 2019 Apr 24;14(4):e0214288.

15. Ruggeri P, Lo Monaco L, Musumeci O, Tavilla G, Gaeta M, Caramori G, Toscano A. Ultrasound assessment of diaphragm function in patients with late-onset Pompe disease. *Neurol Sci*. 2020 Aug;41(8):2175–84.

16. Fayssoil A, Behin A, Ogna A, Mompoint D, Amthor H, Clair B, Laforet P, Mansart A, Prigent H, Orlikowski D, Stojkovic T, Vinit S, Carlier R, Eymard B, Lofaso F, Annane D. Diaphragm: Pathophysiology and Ultrasound Imaging in Neuromuscular Disorders. *J Neuromuscul Dis*. 2018;5(1):1–10.

17. Hobson-Webb LD, Simmons Z. Ultrasound in the diagnosis and monitoring of amyotrophic lateral sclerosis: a review. *Muscle Nerve*. 2019 Aug;60(2):114–23.

18. de Carvalho M, Costa J, Swash M. Clinical trials in ALS: a review of the role of clinical and neurophysiological measurements. *Amyotroph Lateral Scler Other Motor Neuron Disord*. 2005 Dec;6(4):202–12.

19. Sartucci F, Pelagatti A, Santin M, Bocci T, Dolciotti C, Bongioanni P. Diaphragm ultrasonography in amyotrophic lateral sclerosis: a diagnostic tool to assess ventilatory dysfunction and disease severity. *Neurol Sci.* 2019 Oct;40(10):2065–71.

20. Yoshioka Y, Ohwada A, Sekiya M, Takahashi F, Ueki J, Fukuchi Y. Ultrasonographic evaluation of the diaphragm in patients with amyotrophic lateral sclerosis. *Respirology.* 2007 Mar;12(2):304–7.

21. Pinto S, Alves P, Pimentel B, Swash M, de Carvalho M. Ultrasound for assessment of diaphragm in ALS. *Clin Neurophysiol.* 2016 Jan;127(1):892–7.

22. Hiwatani Y, Sakata M, Miwa H. Ultrasonography of the diaphragm in amyotrophic lateral sclerosis: clinical significance in assessment of respiratory functions. *Amyotroph Lateral Scler Frontotemporal Degener.* 2013 Mar;14(2):127–31.

23. Zerres K, Rudnik-Schöneborn S, Forrest E, Lusakowska A, Borkowska J, Hausmanowa-Petrusewicz I. A collaborative study on the natural history of childhood and juvenile onset proximal spinal muscular atrophy (type II and III SMA): 569 patients. *J Neurol Sci.* 1997 Feb 27;146(1):67–72.

24. Finkel RS, Mercuri E, Meyer OH, Simonds AK, Schroth MK, Graham RJ, Kirschner J, Iannaccone ST, Crawford TO, Woods S, Muntoni F, Wirth B, Montes J, Main M, Mazzone ES, Vitale M, Snyder B, Quijano-Roy S, Bertini E, Davis RH, Qian Y, Sejersen T; SMA Care group. Diagnosis and management of spinal muscular atrophy: Part 2: Pulmonary and acute care; medications, supplements and immunizations; other organ systems; and ethics. *Neuromuscul Disord.* 2018 Mar;28(3):197–207.

25. Berti B, Buonsenso D, De Rose C, Ferrantini G, De Sanctis R, Forcina N, Mercuri E, Pane M. Point-of-care lung and diaphragm ultrasound in a patient with spinal muscular atrophy with respiratory distress type 1. *J Ultrasound.* 2021 Apr 13.

26. Spiesshoefer J, Henke C, Kabitz HJ, Brix T, Görlich D, Herkenrath S, Randerath W, Young P, Boentert M. The nature of respiratory muscle weakness in patients with late-onset Pompe disease. *Neuromuscul Disord.* 2019 Aug;29(8):618–27.

27. Meng P, Ogna A, Fayssoil A. M Mode Ultrasound and Tissue Doppler Imaging to Assess Diaphragm Feature in Late Onset Pompe Disease. *Neurol Int.* 2020 Nov 13;12(3):55–8.

28. Quijano-Roy S, Khirani S, Colella M, Ramirez A, Aloui S, Wehbi S, de Becdelievre A, Carlier RY, Allamand V, Richard P, Azzi V, Estournet B, Fauroux B. Diaphragmatic dysfunction in Collagen VI myopathies. *Neuromuscul Disord.* 2014 Feb;24(2):125–33.

29. De Antonio M, Dogan C, Daidj F, Eymard B, Puymirat J, Mathieu J, Gagnon C, Katsahian S, Filnemus Myotonic Dystrophy Study Group, Hamroun D, Bassez G. The DM-scope registry: a rare disease innovative framework bridging the gap between research and medical care. *Orphanet J Rare Dis.* 2019 Jun 3;14(1):122.

30. Evangelista MA, Dias FAL, Dourado Júnior MET, do Nascimento GC, Sarmento A, Gualdi LP, Aliverti A, Resqueti V, Fregonezi GAF. Noninvasive assessment of respiratory muscle strength and activity in Myotonic dystrophy. *PLoS One.* 2017 Jun 8;12(6):e0177318.

31. Thil C, Agrinier N, Chenuel B, Poussel M. Longitudinal course of lung function in myotonic dystrophy type 1. *Muscle Nerve.* 2017 Oct;56(4):816–818.

32. Henke C, Spiesshoefer J, Kabitz HJ, Herkenrath S, Randerath W, Brix T, Görlich D, Young P, Boentert M. Characteristics of respiratory muscle involvement in myotonic dystrophy type 1. *Neuromuscul Disord.* 2020 Jan;30(1):17–27.

33. Wohlgemuth M, Horlings CGC, van der Kooi EL, Gilhuis HJ, Hendriks JCM, van der Maarel SM, van Engelen BGM, Heijdra YF, Padberg GW. Respiratory function in facioscapulohumeral muscular dystrophy 1. *Neuromuscul Disord.* 2017 Jun;27(6):526–30.

34. Sacconi S, Briand-Suleau A, Gros M, Baudoin C, Lemmers RJLF, Rondeau S, Lagha N, Nigumann P, Cambieri C, Puma A, Chapon F, Stojkovic T, Vial C, Bouhour F, Cao M, Pegoraro E, Petiot P, Behin A, Marc B, Eymard B, Echaniz-Laguna A, Laforet P, Salviati L, Jeanpierre M, Cristofari G, van der Maarel SM. FSHD1 and FSHD2 form a disease continuum. *Neurology.* 2019 May 7;92(19):e2273-e2285.

35. Scully MA, Eichinger KJ, Donlin-Smith CM, Tawil R, Statland JM. Restrictive lung involvement in facioscapulohumeral muscular dystrophy. *Muscle Nerve.* 2014 Nov;50(5):739–43.

36. Stübgen JP, Schultz C. Lung and respiratory muscle function in facioscapulohumeral muscular dystrophy. *Muscle Nerve.* 2009 Jun;39(6):729–34.

37. Henke C, Spiesshoefer J, Kabitz HJ, Herkenrath S, Randerath W, Brix T, Görlich D, Young P, Boentert M. Respiratory muscle weakness in facioscapulohumeral muscular dystrophy. *Muscle Nerve.* 2019 Dec;60(6):679–86.

38. Fayssoil A, Stojkovic T, Ogna A, Laforet P, Prigent H, Lofaso F, Orlikowski D, Bassez G, Eymard B, Behin A. Assessment of diaphragm motion using ultrasonography in a patient with facio-scapulo-humeral dystrophy: A case report. *Medicine.* 2019 Jan;98(4):e13887.

39. Birnkrant DJ, Bushby K, Bann CM, Alman BA, Apkon SD, Blackwell A, Case LE, Cripe L, Hadjiyannakis S, Olson AK, Sheehan DW, Bolen J, Weber DR, Ward LM; DMD Care Considerations Working Group. Diagnosis and management of Duchenne muscular dystrophy, part 2: respiratory, cardiac, bone health, and orthopaedic management. *Lancet Neurol.* 2018 Apr;17(4):347–61.

40. Laviola M, Priori R, D'Angelo MG, Aliverti A. Assessment of diaphragmatic thickness by ultrasonography in Duchenne muscular dystrophy (DMD) patients. *PLoS One.* 2018 Jul 26;13(7):e0200582.

41. Fayssoil A, Chaffaut C, Ogna A, Stojkovic T, Lamothe L, Mompoint D, Meng P, Prigent H, Clair B, Behin A, Laforet P, Bassez G, Carlier R, Orlikowski D, Amthor H, Quijano Roy S, Crenn P, Chevret S, Eymard B, Lofaso F, Annane D. Echographic assessment of diaphragmatic function in duchenne muscular dystrophy from childhood to adulthood. *J Neuromuscul Dis.* 2019;6(1):55–64.

42. Melacini P, Fanin M, Danieli GA, et al. Cardiac involvement in Becker muscular dystrophy. *J Am Coll Cardiol.* 1993;22:1927–34.

43. Godoy DA, Mello LJ, Masotti L, Di Napoli M. The myasthenic patient in crisis: an update of the management in Neurointensive Care Unit. *Arq Neuropsiquiatr.* 2013 Sep;71(9A):627–39.

44. Juel VC. Myasthenia gravis: management of myasthenic crisis and perioperative care. *Semin Neurol*. 2004 Mar;24(1):75–81.

45. Weinberg M, Cavalcante JA, Choy T, Ahmad S. A 23-year-old man with dyspnea during myasthenia crisis. *Chest*. 2019 Jun;155(6):e155–7.

46. Maskin LP, Wilken M, Rodriguez Lucci F, Wisnivesky JP, Barroso F, Wainsztein N. Risk factors for respiratory failure among hospitalized patients with Guillain-Barré syndrome. *Neurologia*. 2021 May 29:S0213–4853(21)00082–7.

47. Lawn ND, Fletcher DD, Henderson RD, Wolter TD, Wijdicks EF. Anticipating mechanical ventilation in Guillain-Barre syndrome. *Arch Neurol*. 2001 Jun;58(6):893–8.

10

Other Applications of Diaphragm Ultrasound: Trauma, Malignancies, Ultrasound-Guided Procedures

**Annia Schreiber, Cristian Deana,
Luigi Vetrugno, and Massimo Zambon**

Trauma

Diaphragm US in the trauma setting has several applications. For instance, it can be used to identify a direct injury to the diaphragm (as a consequence of a blunt or penetrating trauma of the chest or abdomen), to assess diaphragm excursion, activity, and function following traumatic spinal cord injury (SCI), and to predict the clinical outcome of traumatized patients.

Diaphragm rupture as a consequence of trauma is not a common event; its prevalence ranges from 0.8% to approximately 5% of patients admitted to the emergency department with multiple traumatic injuries (1, 2). However, despite its rarity, it is a serious complication and a delay in diagnosis may result in significant morbidity and mortality (3, 4).

In the case of blunt trauma, the majority of the tears occur in the posterolateral portion of the diaphragm, where the structure is embryologically weaker (5, 6), and on the left side (probably due to a contralateral protective effect of the liver) (7–9). Partially due to its rarity and its anatomical location, and mainly due to the severity of concurrent injuries, the diagnosis of diaphragmatic rupture is sometimes missed, and often delayed (10). This is especially true when radiologic methods, relying on indirect signs of diaphragm rupture (such as herniated abdominal content, elevation of the hemidiaphragm, or visualization of the nasogastric tube in the chest), are used to investigate the diagnostic suspect (10). Ultrasound has previously shown an extremely high sensitivity and high positive predictive value in identifying diaphragm rupture (11). This is thanks to the fact that the technique mainly relies on direct signs, which are also highly specific, as well as some indirect signs. The direct signs include visualization of the disrupted diaphragm itself (frequently associated with bowel herniation), or of a floating torn free edge of the diaphragm (within a body of collected fluid), or the impossibility to visualize the diaphragm. The sensitivity of the technique is further enhanced when indirect signs are also detected. The indirect sonographic findings consist of: the presence of pleural effusion and/or fluid collection in the subphrenic space adjacent to the diaphragm rupture, splenic laceration, concomitant rib fractures, and visualization of the liver/bowel herniating through the diaphragmatic tear (11, 12).

An additional sign of diaphragmatic injury following blunt abdominal trauma – which has, to our knowledge, only been described in relation to computer tomography (CT), but is potentially identifiable by means of US – is an increase in diaphragm thickness (13). This finding has only been described on the same side of the injury, and frequently adjacent to the area of the defect; in some cases, an increase in diaphragm thickness may be the sole sign of injury to this organ. Such thickening (nodular or smooth, focal or diffuse) may depict an area of oedema or hematoma within the muscle rather than an actual muscular rupture or tear (13). However, considering that an increase in thickness has previously been associated with an increased likelihood of diaphragmatic rupture at a later stage, it is highly likely that it points to a susceptible area that deserves monitoring (14).

Less is known about US findings in relation to penetrating trauma. This is probably related to the fact that penetrating diaphragm injuries either tend to be very small, and as a consequence tend to go unidentified, or, more frequently, such patients are subjected to direct emergent laparotomy, and thus the diaphragm is inspected and repaired directly in the surgical setting (15). However, we can speculate that US findings are able to indicate, as other diagnostic techniques are also able to, the trajectory of the penetrating object, which may not be very evident if the penetrating object is very small, especially in the absence of a pressure gradient, which would otherwise force the abdominal contents into the chest (15).

The use of diaphragm US in trauma medicine poses several advantages, including ease of execution, the possibility of real-time imaging in multiple planes, and the possibility of monitoring patients closely before and after surgical repair. Not only do these advantages allow the clinician to identify the entity of a diaphragm tear directly, but they also permit the early detection of pre- or post-operative deteriorations and/or complications in the patient, potentially improving the patient's final outcome. Possible limitations in the visualization of the signs of diaphragm rupture include the presence of gas in the stomach or splenic/hepatic flexure of the colon, subcutaneous emphysema, and chest/abdomen bandages.

In trauma patients suffering from traumatic spinal cord injury (SCI), diaphragm US can be used to assess the activity and function of the diaphragm (and of other muscles, such as parasternal intercostals, sternocleidomastoid, and abdominal muscles), as well as paradoxical upward movement or immobility after injury. It can also be used to monitor the recovery of these symptoms at different time points.

Depending on the level and degree of completeness of the SCI, as well as on the duration of the injury, the movement, activity, and function of the diaphragm may be preserved, temporally impaired due to a condition of spinal shock, or definitively impaired due to denervation (16). Diaphragmatic activity and function can be assessed by US by measuring the thickening fraction (TF_{dia}) during tidal breathing and during maximal inspiratory effort, respectively; diaphragmatic movement can be assessed by measuring excursion in deep unassisted breathing (17).

Compared with healthy subjects, a reduction in TF_{dia}, both during tidal breathing and deep breathing, together with a decrease in pulmonary function tests, was previously found in patients with cervical spine lesions (C2–C5) admitted to a rehabilitation centre (18, 19). Relevant increases in US-measured diaphragmatic thickness were also described in these same patients (18).

An increase in thickness associated with a decrease in TF_{dia} can be related to several factors in patients with traumatic SCI, all of which are worth monitoring with US. In a more acute phase, an increase in diaphragm thickness may occur, as mentioned above, as a consequence of a direct structural injury to the diaphragm (13, 14), or it may result from systemic inflammation in the context of a severe clinical picture (20). At a later stage, and under more stable conditions, it may be due to a caudal shift of the diaphragm (with consequent muscle fibre shortening) in the upright position in patients with a lack of abdominal muscle tone (16). Finally, an increase in diaphragm thickness may reflect muscle hypertrophy following inspiratory muscle training (21). The trend towards a long-term increase in diaphragmatic thickness would seem to be more typical of SCI patients not requiring mechanical ventilation (MV), as was the case in the previously mentioned studies (18, 19). In SCI patients requiring prolonged MV, in analogy with other critically ill patients with no SCI, a progressive reduction in diaphragmatic thickness as an index of atrophy seems more probable (22); however, more evidence is required to confirm this speculation.

The structure, activity, and function of the diaphragm after SCI may be subject to change, either in accordance with the natural history of the spine injury, or as a consequence of interventions, such as respiratory muscle training techniques or diaphragm pacing aimed at improving respiratory function. Monitoring these changes by means of US, as done in mechanically ventilated ICU patients with no SCI (23–25), may allow the clinician to assess readiness to wean and predict weaning outcomes; once again, further trials conducted in this specific patient population are needed to confirm this hypothesis.

Diaphragm US in the context of trauma has also been applied with the aim of identifying, as early as possible, patients with impaired lung function as these patients are at a higher risk of developing complications after trauma. In particular, a study by O'Hara and colleagues found that in adult patients with blunt trauma and more than one rib fracture, as identified by chest computed tomography, US measurements of the diaphragm performed within 48 hours of admission to a level I trauma centre showed the TF_{dia} during tidal breathing to be inversely correlated to the subjects' inspiratory capacity (IC) as measured on a handheld incentive spirometer (26). The opposite relationship is instead typical in healthy subjects (27). Moreover, the study found that maximal TF_{dia} measured during maximal inspiration did not show any significant correlation with IC. Finally, maximal TF_{dia} in rib fracture patients appeared to be lower compared with normal values reported for healthy subjects in the literature. If this latter finding is expected, and if it is also related to the pain experienced by the patient in performing maximal inspiratory manoeuvres, the inverse correlation between IC and tidal TF_{dia} and the absence of a correlation between IC and maximal TF_{dia} are novel and have potentially relevant clinical and pathophysiological implications. Indeed, as suggested by the authors, this could imply that, in the presence of rib fractures, other muscles are recruited to contribute towards increasing the IC. This could reflect a change in the respiratory mechanics and in the physiological interactions between the diaphragm and other respiratory muscles. This hypothesis needs to be confirmed by means of physiological studies that simultaneously assess the activation of different respiratory muscles. Moreover, as none of the patients enrolled in the cited study required MV despite these findings, their possible clinical and prognostic implications need to be extensively explored.

References

1. Cox EF. Blunt abdominal trauma: A five year analysis of 870 patients following celiotomy. Ann Surg. 1984;199(Table 4).

2. Kearney PA, Rouhana SW, Burney RE. Blunt rupture of the diaphragm: Mechanism, diagnosis, and treatment. *Ann Emerg Med*. 1989;18(12):1326–30.

3. Rodriguez-Morales G, Rodriguez A, Shatney CH. Acute rupture of the diaphragm in blunt trauma: analysis of 60 patients. *J Trauma*. 1996;26(5):438–44.

4. Hegarty M, Bryer J, Angorn I, Backer L. Delayed presentation of a traumatic diaphragmatic hernia. *Ann Surg*. 1978;188(2):229–33.

5. Voeller GR, Reisser JR, Fabian TC, Kudsk K, Mangiante EC. Blunt diaphragm injuries. A five-year experience. *Am Surg*. 1990 Jan;56(1):28–31.

6. Lucido JL, Wall CA. Rupture of the diaphragm due to blunt trauma. *New Repub*. 1963;86:989–99.

7. Pipkin NL, Hamit HF. Traumatic perforation of the diaphragm. *South Mediacl J*. 1988;81(11):1347–50.

8. Sukul DMKSK, Kats E, Johannes EJ. Sixty-three cases of traumatic injury of the diaphragm. *Injury*. 1991;22(4):303–6.

9. Shah R, Sabanathan S, Mearns AJ, Choudhury AK. Traumatic rupture of diaphragm. *Ann Thorac Surg*. 1995;60(5):1444–9.

10. Smithers BM, O'Loughlin B, Strong RW. Diagnosis of ruptured diaphragm following blunt trauma: results from 85 cases. *Aust N Z J Surg*. 1991;61(10):737–41.

11. Kim HH, Shin YR, Kim KJ, Hwang SS, Ha HK, Byun JY, et al. Blunt traumatic rupture of the diaphragm: sonographic diagnosis. *J Ultrasound Med*. 1997;16(9):593–8.

12. Somers JM, Gleeson FV., Flower CDR. Rupture of the right hemidiaphragm following blunt trauma: the use of ultrasound in diagnosis. *Clin Radiol*. 1990;42(2):97–101.

13. Leung JC, Nance ML, Schwab CW, Miller WT. Thickening of the diaphragm: a new computer tomography sign of diaphragm injury. *J Thorac Imaging*. 1999;14:126–9.

14. Nchimi A, Szapiro D, Ghaye B, Willems V, Khamis J, Haquet L, et al. Helical CT of blunt diaphragmatic rupture. *Am J Roentgenol*. 2005;184(1):24–30.

15. Hammer MM, Raptis DA, Mellnick VM, Bhalla S, Raptis CA. Traumatic injuries of the diaphragm: overview of imaging findings and diagnosis. *Abdom Radiol*. 2017;42(4):1020–7.

16. Winslow C, Rozovsky J. Effect of spinal cord injury on the respiratory system. *Am J Phys Med Rehabil*. 2003;82(10):803–14.

17. Valette X, Seguin A, Daubin C, Brunet J, Sauneuf B, Terzi N, et al. Diaphragmatic dysfunction at admission in intensive care unit: the value of diaphragmatic ultrasonography. *Intensive Care Med*. 2015;41(3):557–9.

18. Malas FÜ, Köseoğlu F, Kara M, Ece H, Aytekin M, Öztürk GT, et al. Diaphragm ultrasonography and pulmonary function tests in patients with spinal cord injury. *Spinal Cord.* 2019;57(8):679–83.

19. Zhu Z, Li J, Yang D, Du L, Yang M. Ultrasonography of diaphragm can predict pulmonary function in spinal cord injury patients: A pilot case-control study. *Med Sci Monit.* 2019;25:5369–74.

20. Ebihara S, Hussain SNA, Danialou G, Cho WK, Gottfried SB, Petrof BJ. Mechanical ventilation protects against diaphragm injury in sepsis: Interaction of oxidative and mechanical stresses. *Am J Respir Crit Care Med.* 2002;165(2):221–8.

21. West CR, Taylor BJ, Campbell IG, Romer LM. Effects of inspiratory muscle training on exercise responses in Paralympic athletes with cervical spinal cord injury. *Scand J Med Sci Sport.* 2014;24(5):764–72.

22. Goligher EC, Fan E, Herridge MS, Murray A, Vorona S, Brace D, et al. Evolution of diaphragm thickness during mechanical ventilation: Impact of inspiratory effort. *Am J Respir Crit Care Med.* 2015;192(9):1080–8.

23. DiNino E, Gartman EJ, Sethi JM, McCool FD. Diaphragm ultrasound as a predictor of successful extubation from mechanical ventilation. *Thorax.* 2014;69(5):423–7.

24. Ferrari G, De Filippi G, Elia F, Panero F, Volpicelli G, Apra F. Diaphragm ultrasound as a new index of discontinuation from mechanical ventilation. *Crit Ultrasound J.* 2014;6(1):8.

25. Farghaly S, Hasan AA. Australian critical care diaphragm ultrasound as a new method to predict extubation outcome in mechanically ventilated patients. *Aust Crit Care.* 2017;30(1):37–43.

26. O'Hara DN, Randazzo S, Ahmad S, Taub E, Huang E, Vosswinkel JA, et al. Diaphragm ultrasound: a novel approach to assessing pulmonary function in patients with traumatic rib fractures. *J Trauma Acute Care Surg.* 2020;89(1):96–102.

27. Wait JL, Nahormek PA, Yost WT, Rochester DP. Diaphragmatic thickness-lung volume relationship in vivo. *J App Physiol.* 1989;67(4):1560–8.

Malignancies

Lung cancer may be primary (arising from abnormal lung cells) or secondary (metastases originating from other sites in the body). Lung involvement in metastatic cancer is frequent since the lungs form a sort of "filter", being exposed to all circulating cancer cells. However, the lungs are not the sole site for tumour development within the thorax; the pleura, ribs, and mediastinum also present potential locations for cancer formation. The clinical manifestations of thoracic malignancies vary greatly, ranging from asymptomatic tumours to life threatening conditions, such as acute respiratory failure due to tracheal involvement.[1]

Traditional imaging modalities for assessing patients with malignancies in the thorax include chest X-ray, computed tomography scan (CT scan), and in some cases magnetic resonance (MRI). Lung ultrasound can also be used to explore many of the above-mentioned sites of cancerization; it is an easy-to-use bedside tool which in some cases can be considered an alternative to the traditional techniques.[2]

Superficial lung nodules can be biopsied using ultrasound-assisted needle aspiration – a technique proven to be easy, safe, effective, and more cost-effective than other techniques, such as CT-scanning.[3] This technique has also been implemented during video-assisted thoracoscopic surgery (VATS) for lung metastasis resection.[4]

Pleural thickenings in need of characterization might also be studied using ultrasound; for example, lesion elasticity assessed by transthoracic shear wave ultrasound is a valuable tool, in addition to CT and grayscale ultrasound, for differentiating between benign and malignant tissue and can be used to guide the biopsy of peripheral subpleural lung lesions.[5] In addition to the standard B-mode examination, colour doppler can help physicians rule in or out a malignant pleural plaque, which commonly appear as a thickening of the pleural line exceeding 1 cm.[6]

Another consequence of cancer in the thorax that may be identified during diagnostic work-up is diaphragm paralysis due to phrenic nerve involvement. The diaphragm has increasingly become the subject of study in the ICU over recent years due to its prominent role in patients undergoing mechanical ventilation.[7] Diaphragm weakness is a frequent cause of respiratory failure in the ICU, and diaphragm function can be studied using ultrasound.[8]

The diaphragm is innervated by the phrenic nerve, which is approachable with ultrasound especially in its cervical portion. Some lung neoplasms, such as Pancoast tumours, invade the structures near the apex of the lung, including the phrenic nerve. This results in hemidiaphragm paralysis, with the possibility of respiratory failure.[9]

In the case of pleural effusions (PLEFF), since this fluid always originates from the lung or pleura, a small amount of the fluid collected during pleural drainage should always be sent to a pathology laboratory for cytological analysis so that any neoplastic cells within the fluid can be identified as soon as possible.

Rib fractures also have the potential to become a site of secondary neoplasms, as in the case of lung, prostate, or breast cancer. Rib fractures, especially in children, can be diagnosed by means of ultrasound; it is also possible in adults, except in the case of unfavourable anatomy, such as obesity.[10]

Anomalies within the lung, pleural, or chest wall suspected of neoplasms should also be studied by CT-scan; however, ultrasound can aid the biopsy of these lesions if localized near the pleural line.

References

1. Nasim F, Sabath BF, Eapen GA. Lung cancer. *Med Clin North Am.* 2019 May;103(3):463–473. doi: 10.1016/j.mcna.2018.12.006. PMID: 30955514.

2. Miles MJ, Islam S. Point of care ultrasound in thoracic malignancy. *Ann Transl Med.* 2019 Aug;7(15):350. doi: 10.21037/atm.2019.05.53. PMID: 31516896; PMCID: PMC6712247.

3. Livi V, Paioli D, Cancellieri A, Betti S, Natali F, Ferrari M, Fiorentino M, Trisolini R. Diagnosis and molecular profiling of lung cancer by percutaneous ultrasound-guided biopsy of superficial metastatic sites is safe and highly effective. *Respiration.* 2021 Apr 7:1–8. doi: 10.1159/000514316. Epub ahead of print. PMID: 33827098.

4. Londero F, Castriotta L, Grossi W, Masullo G, Morelli A, Tetta C, Livi U, Maessen JG, Gelsomino S. VATS-US1: thoracoscopic ultrasonography for the identification of

nodules during lung metastasectomy. *Future Oncol.* 2020 Feb;16(5):85–89. doi: 10.2217/fon-2019-0608. Epub 2020 Jan 9. PMID: 31916464.

5. Verschakelen JA. Transthoracic shear wave ultrasound: a noninvasive tool to differentiate between benign and malignant subpleural lung lesions. Eur Respir J. 2021 Mar 25;57(3):2004260. doi: 10.1183/13993003.04260-2020. PMID: 33767002.

6. Dietrich CF, Mathis G, Cui XW, Ignee A, Hocke M, Hirche TO. Ultrasound of the pleurae and lungs. *Ultrasound Med Biol.* 2015 Feb;41(2):351–65. doi: 10.1016/j.ultrasmedbio.2014.10.002. PMID: 25592455.

7. McCool FD, Tzelepis GE. Dysfunction of the diaphragm. *N Engl J Med.* 2012 Mar 8;366(10):932–42. doi: 10.1056/NEJMra1007236. Erratum in: *N Engl J Med.* 2012 May 31;366(22):2138. PMID: 22397655.

8. Vetrugno L, Guadagnin GM, Barbariol F, Langiano N, Zangrillo A, Bove T. Ultrasound imaging for diaphragm dysfunction: a narrative literature review. *J Cardiothorac Vasc Anesth.* 2019 Sep;33(9):2525–2536. doi: 10.1053/j.jvca.2019.01.003. Epub 2019 Jan 4. PMID: 30686657.

9. Kokatnur L, Rudrappa M. Diaphragmatic palsy. *Diseases.* 2018 Feb 13;6(1):16. doi: 10.3390/diseases6010016. PMID: 29438332; PMCID: PMC5871962.

10. Çelik A, Akoglu H, Omercikoglu S, Bugdayci O, Karacabey S, Kabaroglu KA, Onur O, Denizbasi A. The diagnostic accuracy of ultrasonography for the diagnosis of rib fractures in patients presenting to emergency department with blunt chest trauma. *J Emerg Med.* 2021 Jan;60(1):90–97. doi: 10.1016/j.jemermed.2020.06.063. Epub 2020 Nov 18. PMID: 33218837.

Ultrasound-Guided Procedures

Most of the more frequent invasive procedures are nowadays performed with the help of echography. This bedside tool allows for the reduction of procedure-related complications, such as pneumothorax or organ lesions related to invasive manoeuvres. Recently, diaphragmatic ultrasound has shown its utility in several procedures.

Guidance for Needle EMG

Electromyographic examination of the diaphragm can be challenging due to the risk of injury to the lung, liver, spleen, and colon. Ultrasound, providing excellent visualization of nerves and tissues, enhances safety by avoiding accidental needle puncture of vital organs (1). Furthermore, confirmation of needle placement within the diaphragm by direct visualization is particularly helpful in patients with a paralyzed or severely atrophic diaphragm, where the normal sound of motor unit potential firing cannot be relied on to confirm appropriate placement (see reference 2→ video URL). The transducer is placed at the anterior axillary line and rotated so that it is parallel to the intercostal space, typically between the eighth and ninth ribs. The needle is then inserted and advanced in-plane with the transducer, until it can be seen entering the diaphragm. In high-risk patients such as those on anticoagulants or with bleeding disorders, hematoma formation can be visualized immediately, allowing the examiner to terminate the examination or to intervene promptly if clinically indicated.

Assessment of Phrenic Nerve Pacing

Diaphragmatic pacing is a second-line therapy for ventilatory failure due to bilateral paralysis or severe paresis of the diaphragm (3). This population of patients has traditionally been ventilated invasively with a mechanical ventilator, or non-invasively with positive pressure support. However, diaphragmatic pacing can be used in a select group of patients who cannot tolerate, have a desire to be liberated from, or have a desire to delay the need for non-invasive or invasive ventilatory support. Recently, temporary transvenous diaphragm pacing has been tested for ICU patients with Ventilator Induced Diaphragmatic Dysfunction (VIDD) (4). Ultrasound can be useful to obtain information regarding the motion of the diaphragm in patients who are potential candidates for phrenic nerve pacing or to monitor the effect of pacing on the muscle (4, 5).

Assessment of Paralysis after Interscalene Brachial Plexus Block

Interscalene brachial plexus block (ISBPB) is one of the most reliable and commonly performed techniques for regional anaesthesia of the upper extremity. It anaesthetizes the caudal portion of the cervical plexus (C3, C4) and the superior (C5, C6) and middle (C7) trunks of the brachial plexus. The most common complication is phrenic nerve palsy (6, 7). The phrenic nerve arises chiefly from the C4 root, with variable contributions from C3 and C5, it courses caudally between the ventral surface of the anterior scalene muscle and prevertebral fascial layer that covers this muscle, therefore separated from the brachial plexus only by a thin fascial layer. As a result, its block in ISBPB can be explained by the proximity to the brachial plexus or to the cephalad spread of local anaesthetic to the C3–5 roots of the cervical plexus before their formation of the phrenic nerve.

Phrenic nerve block is associated with significant reductions in ventilatory function, and potentially serious complications can affect patients with limited pulmonary reserve such as those with chronic obstructive pulmonary disease (COPD), the morbidly obese, or the elderly.

In these patients, ultrasound allows early identification of diaphragmatic hemi-paresis, helps to plan an adequate monitoring, and allows to provide a safer post-operative course.

References

1. Boon AJ, Alsharif KI, Harper CM, Smith J. Ultrasound-guided needle EMG of the diaphragm: technique description and case report. *Muscle Nerve* 2008 Dec;38(6):1623–6.

2. https://movementdisorders.onlinelibrary.wiley.com/page/journal/23301619/homepage/mdc313043-sup-v001.htm

3. Glenn WW, Hogan JF, Loke JS, Ciesielski TE, Phelps ML, Rowedder R. Ventilatory support by pacing of the conditioned diaphragm in quadriplegia. *N Engl J Med* 1984 May 3;310:1150–5.doi: 10.1056/NEJM198405033101804.

4. Evans, D., Shure, D., Clark, L., et al. Temporary transvenous diaphragm pacing vs. standard of care for weaning from mechanical ventilation: study protocol for a randomized trial. *Trials* 2019;20:60. doi: 10.1186/s13063-018-3171-9

5. Skalsky AJ, Lesser DJ, McDonald CM. Evaluation of phrenic nerve and diaphragm function with peripheral nerve stimulation and M-mode ultrasonography in potential pediatric phrenic nerve or diaphragm pacing candidates. *Phys Med Rehabil Clin N Am* 2015 Feb;26:133–43. doi: 10.1016/j.pmr.2014.09.010. PMID: 25479785

6. Urmey WF, Talts KH, Sharrock NE. One hundred percent incidence of hemidiaphragmatic paresis associated with interscalene brachial plexus anesthesia as diagnosed by ultrasonography. *Anesth Analg* 1991;72:498–503.

7. Urmey, William F., McDonald, Marianne BS. RRT hemidiaphragmatic paresis during interscalene brachial plexus block. *Anesth Analg* 1992;74:352–357.

8. Effect of local anaesthetic volume (20 vs 5 ml) on the efficacy and respiratory consequences of ultrasound-guided interscalene brachial plexus block.

Part IV

New Perspectives

11

Ultrasound Assessment of the Accessory Respiratory Muscles

Myrte Wennen, Annemijn H. Jonkman, Zhonghua Shi, and Pieter R. Tuinman

Introduction

Ultrasound is a useful and increasingly popular bedside technique for assessing respiratory muscle function in critically ill patients [1]. Although it is mainly employed to assess the diaphragm, ultrasound evaluation of the accessory respiratory muscles is gaining interest [2–5]. The respiratory muscle pump is a complex system consisting of various muscles that closely work together in breathing. In tidal breathing, only the diaphragm and external intercostal muscles are active [6–8]. In case of high inspiratory or expiratory respiratory demand, for example, due to chronic obstructive pulmonary disease (COPD), degenerative muscle diseases, or acute respiratory failure, the load on the diaphragm increases and as a response, accessory respiratory muscles are recruited.

DOI: 10.1201/9781003128694-15

Extra-diaphragmatic inspiratory muscles consist of the external intercostal, parasternal intercostal, pectoralis, scalene, and sternocleidomastoid muscle. Recruitment of these muscles was shown to be dependent on diaphragm weakness [9–11]. For example, in mechanically ventilated patients an inverse correlation was found between parasternal muscle thickening fraction and pressure generating capacity of the diaphragm [12]. Decreased thickness of the intercostal muscles was associated with prolonged mechanical ventilation and ICU length of stay [13]. However, evidence is still very limited.

The main expiratory muscles include the lateral abdominal wall muscles, consisting of the external oblique (EO), internal oblique (IO) and transverse abdominis (TrA) muscle, and the rectus abdominis (RA), which are mainly active during forced expiration [6, 14–16]. The expiratory muscles are recruited with high inspiratory loading, increased end-expiratory lung volume, and low inspiratory muscle capacity [14, 17]. Expiratory muscles are recruited in patients with weaning failure, probably due to increased respiratory demand and/or diaphragm weakness [17]. Additionally, weakness of the expiratory muscles is also associated with worse weaning outcomes [18], probably due to decreased cough strength [19].

Examination of the extra-diaphragmatic inspiratory and expiratory muscles by ultrasound adds complementary information in the evaluation of patient respiratory effort (recruitment, respective contribution in the work of breathing, asynchrony) and muscle function, and can help the clinician to detect patients at risk for weaning failure. In this chapter, we provide a structured approach for assessing the accessory respiratory muscles by ultrasound, including ultrasound-derived parameters such as thickness and thickening fraction (TF) and their normal values (if known). We also discuss limitations, potential clinical applications, and future developments for functional imaging.

Ultrasound Techniques

A linear 10–15 MHz ultrasound probe is used for visualizing the parasternal intercostal muscle and abdominal wall muscles, similar to the diaphragm. This type of probe is suitable for identifying superficial structures and as such has a good near-field resolution. At all times, the probe should be kept perpendicular to the skin and minimal pressure to the skin should be applied to avoid muscle deformation.

Parasternal Intercostal Muscle Ultrasonography

With the patient in supine or semi-recumbent position, the probe is placed perpendicular to the anterior thoracic surface in the sagittal plane, at the level of the second and third intercostal space, 3–5 cm laterally from the sternum [20], although for certain cases 6–8 cm may be required [12]. In B-mode, the muscle can be identified as the biconcave structure between two hyperechoic fascia attached to the ribs, which appear as dark, hypoechoic ovals (see Figure 11.1). Beneath the parasternal intercostal muscle, the pleural line is visible and on top lies the pectoral muscle. The thickening fraction of the intercostal muscles (TFic) can be computed as the percentage of increase in muscle thickness during inspiration using the end inspiratory thickness (Tei) and end expiratory thickness (Tee) of the parasternal intercostal muscle: $\text{TFic} = \left(\left(\text{Tei} - \text{Tee} \right) / \text{Tee} \right) \times 100\%$. Tee and Tei are measured from M-mode imaging

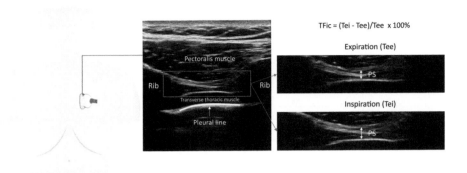

Figure 11.1 Probe position and example ultrasound images of the parasternal intercostal muscle. *PS = parasternal intercostal muscle, TFic = thickening fraction of the intercostal muscle, Tei = end-inspiratory thickness, Tee = end-expiratory thickness*

or B-mode video/frames with the markers placed within the inner borders of the fascia. It is recommended to measure an average value of at least three separate breaths.

Table 11.1 lists available reference values of thickness and thickening fraction of the parasternal intercostal muscle. Dres et al. (2020) reported a median thickening fraction of 3% (interquartile range (IQR): 2–5%) in healthy subjects at rest and 5% (IQR: 3–8) vs. 17% (IQR: 10–25) in ICU patients without and with diaphragm dysfunction, respectively [12].

Expiratory Abdominal Muscle Ultrasonography

With the patient in supine position and using B-mode, the EO, IO, and TrA can best be visualized with the probe positioned transverse on the anterior axillary line, midway between the inferior side of the rib cage and iliac crest (see Figure 11.2). These three muscles lie parallel in the ultrasound image with TrA at the bottom, IO in the middle, and EO lies most superficial. The RA muscle can be visualized by positioning the probe 2–3 cm above the umbilicus and 2–3 cm away from the midline (see Figure 11.2). It can be identified as the structure between two fascia, seen as hyperechoic lines. When starting with imaging the RA, the lateral abdominal muscles (EO, IO, and TrA) can easily be found by slowly moving the probe laterally towards the anterior axillary line. Generally, RA is the thickest structure, followed by IO, EO, and TrA (see Figure 11.2) [25].

Using M-mode imaging or a B-mode video of the respiratory cycle, the thickness at end-inspiration (Tei) and end-expiration (Tee) can be measured by placing markers within the inner borders of the fascia. Thickening fraction of the abdominal muscle (TFab) can then be determined as: $TFab = \left(\left(Tee - Tei\right) / Tei\right) \times 100\%$. It should be noted that the TFab quantifies thickening of the expiratory muscles during expiration, while TFic describes thickening during inspiration. Again, it is recommended to measure an average value of at least three separate breaths. The thickening fraction can be measured during unassisted and assisted breathing to identify recruitment of expiratory muscles, indicating an increased load and/or decreased diaphragm capacity.

Table 11.2 summarizes reference values for the thickness of the abdominal muscles with the patient in supine and sitting positions based on and adapted from the review by Tuinman et al. (2020) [1].

Table 11.1 Reference values of thickness and thickening fraction of the parasternal intercostal muscle in the healthy population, COPD patients and ICU patients receiving pressure support ventilation. Values reported as mean (95% CI) or mean ± standard deviation. In not specified, population consisted of both genders. IS = intercostal space, COPD = chronic obstructive pulmonary disease, ICU = intensive care unit, PS = pressure support, Ref. = Reference

		Thickness (mm)	Thickening fraction (%)	Ref.
Healthy population	End-expiration	All: 2.8 (2.1 – 3.3) Men: 3.3 (2.6 – 3.8) Women: 2.2 (2.0 – 2.8) 3.6 ± 0.3		[12] [21]
	End-inspiration	All: 2.8 (2.1 – 3.4) Men: 3.3 (2.8 – 3.9) Women: 2.2 (1.9 – 2.8) 3.7 ± 0.3		[12] [21]
	Mean of end-expiration and end-inspiration	Men: 2.2 ± 0.8 (2nd IS, resting breathing) Men: 2.6 ± 1.0 (2nd IS, maximal breathing)		[22]
			All: 3 (3 – 5) Men: 3 (2 – 5) Women: 3 (0 – 5)	[12]
COPD patients	End-inspiration	4.2 (3.3 – 5.4)		[23]
ICU patients (PS)	End-expiration	4.1 ± 0.7 4.0 (3.1 – 5.0) (normal diaphragm function) 3.9 (3.2 – 5.2) (diaphragm dysfunction)		[24] [12]
	End-inspiration	4.2 ± 0.7 4.2 (3.3 – 5.4) (normal diaphragm function) 4.8 (3.9 – 6.2) (diaphragm dysfunction)		[24] [12]
			2.1 ± 1.7 (normal diaphragm function) 12.7 ± 9.1 (diaphragm dysfunction) 5 (3 – 8) (normal diaphragm function) 17 (10 – 15) (diaphragm dysfunction)	[24] [12]

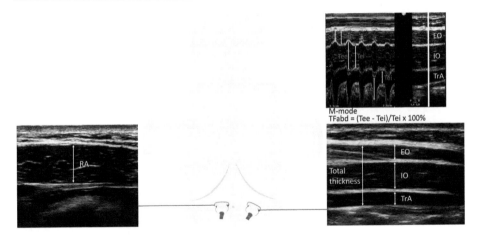

Figure 11.2 Probe position and example images in abdominal wall ultrasound. Left: B-mode ultrasound image of the RA muscle. Bottom right: B-mode ultrasound image of the lateral abdominal muscles. Top right: M-mode ultrasound image of the lateral abdominal muscles, which can be used to compute thickening fraction. *RA = rectus abdominis, EO = external oblique, IO = internal oblique, TrA = transversus abdominis, TFabd = thickening fraction of the abdominal muscles, Tei = end-inspiratory thickness, Tee = end-expiratory thickness*

Tips, Tricks, and Challenges

Ultrasound imaging of the accessory respiratory muscles is a new and simple way to assess the respiratory muscle pump in mechanically ventilated patients, but the application of this technique is still in its infancy. Thickness of the parasternal intercostal muscle and abdominal wall muscles has been studied in healthy subjects as well as critically ill patients (see Tables 11.1 and 11.2). Although thickening fraction may be used to evaluate recruitment of the accessory respiratory muscles, it remains unknown how these values relate to functional parameters such as generated pressures or electrical activity of the muscles (see paragraph **Potential Clinical Applications**). Furthermore, several factors can have a large impact on the measurement of thickness and thickening fraction, such as probe and patient position, placement of measurement markers, but also lung volume and movement of surrounding organs.

Tips and Tricks

The thickness of the accessory respiratory muscles may change during the respiratory cycle [30], and thus measurements are required at both end-inspiration and end-expiration. For the accessory inspiratory muscles, expiration is the resting position and vice versa for the expiratory abdominal muscles. Secondly, it should be kept in mind that the position of the patient affects abdominal muscle thickness [31, 32]. For consecutive measurements, this position should be kept constant and in case of abdominal muscle ultrasound, a supine position of the patient is advised. Marking the probe position on the skin is recommended to reduce variation within measurements originating from changes in probe position. Thirdly, thickness measurements should always be performed in between the hyperechoic fascia and perpendicular to the muscle fibres to accurately measure muscle tissue thickness. In both the

Table 11.2 Reference values of thickness of the abdominal muscles. Values are reported as mean ± standard deviation or median [interquartile range]. If not specified, the population consisted of both genders. Table copied from Tuinman et al. (2020) with permission.

	Abdominal muscles	Reference values thickness	Ref.
General populations	During		
	Sitting, resting		
	External Oblique	7.22 ± 0.91	[26]
		5.5 ± 0.17	[27]
	Internal Oblique	11.48 ± 2.71	[26]
		11.1 ± 3.8	[27]
	Transversus Abdominis	4.62 ± 0.97	[26]
		5.8 ± 1.3	[27]
	Rectus Abdominis	11.0 ± 4.3	[26]
	Supine, resting		
	External Oblique	Men: 6.7 ± 1.7 (R); 6.9 ± 1.6 (L)	[28]
		Women: 5.9 ± 1.8(R); 5.8 ± 1.6(L)*	[25]
		Men: 9.7 ± 2.3(R); 9.6 ± 2.1 (L)	
		Women: 7.3 ± 2.0(R); 7.4 ± 1.5(L)	
		Men: 5.7 ± 1.2 (R); 5.4 ± 1.3 (L)	
		Women: 4.8 ± 1.1(R); 4.8 ± 1.1(L)	
	Internal Oblique	Men: 10.2 ± 2.7(R); 10.4 ± 2.7(L)	[28]
		Women: 7.5 ± 1.8(R); 7.3 ± 1.8(L)*	[25]
		Men: 11.8 ± 2.7(R); 11.7 ± 2.8(L)	
		Women: 8.5 ± 2.2(R); 8.1 ± 2.3(L)	
		Men: 8.9 ± 2.3(R); 8.5 ± 2.0(L)	
		Women: 6.1 ± 1.3(R); 5.8 ± 1.2(L)	
	Transversus Abdominis	Men: 5.4 ± 1.1(R); 5.7 ± 1.1(L)	[28]
		Women: 3.9 ± 0.08(R); 4.4 ± 0.08(L)*	[25]
		Men: 4.5 ± 1.3(R); 5.1 ± 1.3(L)	[29]
		Women: 3.6 ± 0.09(R); 3.7 ± 0.10(L)	
		Men: 4.5 ± 0.09(R); 3.8 ± 0.1(L)	
		Women: 3.5 ± 0.08(R); 3.3 ± 0.07(L)	
		4.7 ± 1.1 (Dominant side); 4.6 ± 0.9 (Non dominant side)	
		Men: 5.0 ± 0.9	
		Women: 4.2 ± 0.7	
	Total thickness of lateral three layers	Men: 34.8 ± 5.9(R); 35.3 ± 6.1(L)	[28]
		Women:27.6 ± 4.4(R); 27.8 ± 4.0(L)*	[29]
		Men: 38.6 ± 6.4(R); 38.8 ± 6.7(L)	
		Women: 29.6 ± 4.6(R); 29.4 ± 4.3(L)	
		21.5 ± 5.9(Dominant side); 20.9 ± 5.5 (Non dominant side)	
		Men: 25.3 ± 3.9	
		Women: 16.6 ± 3.1	
	Rectus Abdominis	Men: 12.5 ± 2.2(R); 12.4 ± 2.4(L)	[28]
		Women:10.2 ± 1.6(R); 10.2 ± 1.5(L)	[25]
		Men: 10.3 ± 1.8(R); 10.4 ± 1.9(L)	
		Women:8.7 ± 1.2(R); 8.3 ± 1.3(L)	
	Supine, contracted		
	Transversus Abdominis	8.7 ± 2.1 (Dominant side); 8.6 ± 2.2 (Non dominant side)	[29]
		Men: 9.8 ± 2.0	
		Women: 7.4 ± 1.2	
	Total thickness of lateral three layers	26.5 ± 8.0 (Dominant side); 26.0 ± 8.2 (Non dominant side)	[29]
		Men: 31.7 ± 6.3	
		Women: 20.0 ± 3.8	
ICU patients	Total thickness of lateral three layers	13.1 [10.2 – 16.1]	[30]

*Measurements performed immediately below the ribcage in the direction vertical alignment with the anterior superior iliac spine.

intercostal and the abdominal wall muscles, the muscle fibres are not always parallel to the skin surface. To overcome this, B-mode may be preferred over M-mode, because in B-mode the markers can be placed in every desired orientation. Fourthly, as mentioned before, when measuring thickness, it is essential to apply minimal probe pressure to the skin to prevent muscle deformations which could affect the measurement.

Additionally, in expiratory muscle ultrasound the separate abdominal wall muscles can move in multiple directions and thereby directly influence thickness and position of adjacent muscle layers. It is therefore recommended to assess the total abdominal muscle thickness (see Figure 11.2) when evaluating changes in expiratory muscle thickness during mechanical ventilation, as was done recently by Shi et al. (2021) [33]. Secondly, one should keep in mind that changes in thickness of the expiratory muscles during respiration may be either a result of active contraction during expiration, or passive lengthening and shortening due to the motion of abdominal contents with respiration.

Reliability and Accuracy

One of the suggested limitations of respiratory muscles ultrasound is its reproducibility. Several factors can affect measurements, such as probe orientation, angle of insonation, and the applied pressure of the transducer to the skin.

In addition, measurements may be more challenging to perform reliably in thinner muscles. The axial resolution of ultrasound using a linear transducer at relatively high frequencies (10–15 MHz) is around 0.10–0.15 mm [5]. This is of particular importance for the parasternal intercostal muscle because the resolution may comprise up to 5.3% (0.15/2.8 * 100, with 2.8 the average thickness (mm), as described in Table 11.1) of its thickness measurements. Considering thickening fractions of, for example, 2.1% (see Table 11.2, no diaphragm dysfunction), this deviation can have considerable impact.

The reproducibility of ultrasound measurements of the parasternal intercostal muscle has been described with an ICC ranging from fair to excellent: 0.65–0.96 and 0.60–0.92 for intra- and inter-observer reproducibility of thickness measurements, respectively [12, 22, 23]. Additionally, Diab et al. (1998) suggested that measurement of the area of the intercostal muscle was more reliable at maximal inhalation compared to exhalation [34]. For thickening fraction, Dres et al. (2020) found an ICC of 0.77 [12].

Several studies report good to excellent intra- and inter-observer reproducibility of static thickness measurements of the abdominal muscles. ICC ranged from 0.76 to 0.99 and 0.75 to 1.0 for intra- and inter-observer reproducibility, respectively [35–38]. In a recent study that evaluated the total thickness of the three lateral abdominal muscles in mechanically ventilated ICU patients, the intra- and inter-observer reproducibility was 0.99 for two raters [30]. Although the ICC was excellent in this study, the range in 95% limits of agreement between observers was relatively wide (–13.1% to 6.8%).

Potential Clinical Applications

Ultrasound of the accessory respiratory muscles in addition to diaphragm ultrasound is helpful for evaluating the respiratory muscle pump as a whole and for assessing potentially increased respiratory efforts. Depending on the clinical question, it can be applied to evaluate anatomic changes over time or to assess muscle recruitment at a certain time point, such as before or during a spontaneous breathing trial (SBT). It can therefore provide insight into the progression of the weakness of the respiratory muscle pump or in possible risk factors for difficult weaning. In general, we suggest performing accessory respiratory muscle ultrasound in concert with other ultrasound measurements. For example, the ABCDE ultrasound approach proposed by Tuinman et al. (2020) was developed to structurally assess the extra-diaphragmatic muscles, together with diaphragm, lung, and cardiac ultrasound in weaning failure patients [1].

Changes in Thickness

Similar to atrophy of the diaphragm, a decrease in thickness of both the internal and external intercostal muscles in patients receiving controlled mechanical ventilation was associated with prolonged duration of mechanical ventilation and increased length of ICU stay [13]. In that study, thickness of the intercostal muscles was measured at the zone of apposition of the diaphragm, i.e., approximately between the mid-axillary and antero-axillary line at the eighth to eleventh intercostal space. Although we propose a different probe position for a structured ultrasound approach, their study demonstrates that monitoring the thickness of the parasternal intercostal muscle may provide insight into development of critical illness-associated respiratory muscle dysfunction.

In COPD patients, thickness of the parasternal intercostal muscle correlated weakly but significantly (r = 0.33) with the percentage of predicted forced expiratory volume in 1 second (FEV1%) [23]. In a consecutive study, it was shown that reduction in residual volume due to endobronchial valve placement negatively correlated with thickness of the parasternal intercostal muscle in these patients [39]. Thickness measurements of the accessory respiratory muscles may thus provide insight into COPD disease severity or progression.

Shi et al. (2021) showed that the total thickness of the lateral abdominal wall muscles decreases by 22%, increases by 12%, and remains stable in 66% of critically ill patients within the first week of mechanical ventilation, with changes in thickness defined as a change of > 15% (increase or decrease) from baseline thickness [30]. Remarkably, the increase in muscle thickness was mostly due to thickening of the fascia and not of the muscular tissue. In critically ill children, expiratory muscle thickness rapidly changed (with > 10%) within four days after intubation with an increase in thickness in 20% and a decrease in 44% of children [35]. Interestingly, in both of these studies [30, 35], changes in expiratory muscle thickness were not associated with changes in diaphragm thickness, indicating a different response of these muscles to mechanical ventilation and critical illness. This response, as well as reference values for (clinically relevant changes in) thickness, should be further studied.

Recruitment of Accessory Respiratory Muscles

Recent studies indicate that parasternal intercostal muscle thickening fraction is an important finding in mechanically ventilated patients; Dres et al. (2020) found a higher thickening fraction in patients who failed an SBT compared to patients who succeeded in an SBT (TFic of 18% vs. 7% for SBT failure vs. success) and in patients with diaphragm dysfunction compared to those without (TFic of 17% versus 5% for patients with vs. without diaphragm dysfunction) [12]. Secondly, the level of pressure support was shown to be negatively associated with parasternal intercostal muscle thickening fraction [12, 24]. Similarly, abdominal muscle ultrasound can be used to assess enhanced expiratory muscle efforts in mechanically ventilated patients [14], as recruitment of these muscles has been described in patients failing a weaning trial [17]. In addition, an increase in thickness of the TrA was strongly correlated with its electrical activity [40] and with the gastric pressure developed during an expiratory manoeuvre [27]. However, these studies [27, 40] were performed in healthy subjects, making translation of findings to the ICU setting yet limited. The complex interaction between the different abdominal wall muscles, with individual layers activating and thickening in different directions according to their fibre orientation, and their correlation with functional parameters (e.g., electrical activity or pressure) should be studied more thoroughly in critically ill patients.

Novel Techniques and Future Research Questions

In the last decades, technological advances have allowed researchers and clinicians to use ultrasound for functional imaging and quantification of elastic properties. Applications that are currently studied for the diaphragm include strain imaging, shear wave elastography, and echogenicity [41–43]. These techniques, which are already widely applied in cardiac imaging, aim at quantifying tissue properties and function of the muscle and could thus be interesting techniques to explore for evaluating the accessory respiratory muscles, since changes in muscle stiffness and deformation can reflect alterations in muscle physiology.

Strain Imaging

Strain imaging computes the deformation of tissue by tracking speckles over time. Although seen as noise in conventional echograms, speckles are an excellent feature to quantify the motion and deformation of structures, allowing measurements of displacement and deformation in two directions. This is especially of interest for the abdominal wall muscles, because they have more degrees of freedom compared to the diaphragm.

Shear Wave Elastography

Shear wave elastography is used to define tissue stiffness as quantified by its elastic modulus. Both tissue deformation and stiffness may be related to muscle function, as was demonstrated for the diaphragm in healthy volunteers [41, 44] and ICU patients [45], where deformation and diaphragm shear modulus during inspiration were associated with (changes in) transdiaphragmatic pressure. Therefore, shear wave elastography might offer a new non-invasive method for gauging diaphragm effort, which could be an interesting application for other respiratory muscles as well [41]. The technique has been successfully performed for the abdominal muscles of healthy controls and patients suffering from scoliosis and incisional hernia after laparotomy [46, 47], but not in accessory inspiratory muscles.

Echogenicity

Echogenicity could also be a parameter of interest in ultrasound of the accessory respiratory muscles. Echogenicity is measured using a histogram of a region of interest within the muscle and could provide a measure of muscle quality. Increased muscle echogenicity has been suggested to reflect muscle injury or degeneration, as validated in muscle biopsies in humans and rats [48, 49]. Dependence on the ultrasound settings is one of the main limitations of this measurement, since changes in, e.g., gain or depth directly influence grey values of the muscle within the ultrasound image [50]. In mechanically ventilated patients, measurement of echogenicity of the diaphragm was reported as reproducible and feasible; echogenicity increased in over one-third of the patients during the course of mechanical ventilation [51]. Wallbridge et al. (2018) performed echogenicity measurements in the parasternal intercostal muscle and found a moderate, negative correlation (r = −0.32) between echogenicity and FEV1% predicted, although the measurements were quite variable for different probe positions (e.g., left–right or second and third intercostal space). Future research is needed to further evaluate the use of echogenicity measurements in the accessory respiratory muscles.

Conclusion

Ultrasound imaging of the respiratory muscles is a valuable tool in clinical practice: it is non-invasive, easy to learn, relatively cheap, and can be used bed-side. Although ultrasound is already indispensable in evaluating function and aspects of the diaphragm, its use for the accessory respiratory muscles is sometimes overlooked. In this chapter, we provide a structured approach for performing ultrasound of the accessory respiratory muscles in clinical practice. Although implementation of this technique is still at an early stage, mastery of the technique could provide the clinician with important information on the complete respiratory muscle pump. Eventually, this may aid in identifying patients at risk for development of respiratory muscle dysfunction or screen for potential risk factors of weaning failure.

References

1. P. Tuinman et al., "Respiratory muscle ultrasonography: methodology, basic and advanced principles and clinical applications in ICU and ED patients: a narrative review," *Intensive Care Medicine*, vol. 46, no. 01/14, p. 594–605, 2020.

2. B.-P. Dubé and M. Dres, "Diaphragm dysfunction: diagnostic approaches and management strategies," (in eng), *Journal of Clinical Medicine*, vol. 5, no. 12, p. 113, 2016.

3. E. C. Goligher et al., "Evolution of diaphragm thickness during mechanical ventilation. Impact of inspiratory effort," *American Journal of Respiratory and Critical Care Medicine*, vol. 192, no. 9, pp. 1080–1088, 2015/11/01 2015.

4. L. M. A. Heunks, J. Doorduin, and J. G. van der Hoeven, "Monitoring and preventing diaphragm injury," *Current Opinion in Critical Care*, vol. 21, no. 1, pp. 34–41, 2015.

5. M. Haaksma, P. R. Tuinman, and L. Heunks, "Ultrasound to assess diaphragmatic function in the critically ill-a critical perspective," *Annals of Translational Medicine*, vol. 5, no. 5, p. 114, Mar 2017.

6. A. De Troyer and A. M. Boriek, "Mechanics of the respiratory muscles," *Comprehensive Physiology*, pp. 1273–1300, 2011/07/01 2011. https://doi.org/10.1002/cphy.c100009

7. A. De Troyer, P. A. Kirkwood, and T. A. Wilson, "Respiratory action of the intercostal muscles," *Physiological Reviews*, vol. 85, no. 2, pp. 717–756, 2005/04/01 2005.

8. A. De Troyer, A. Legrand, P. A. Gevenois, and T. A. Wilson, "Mechanical advantage of the human parasternal intercostal and triangularis sterni muscles," (in eng), *Journal of Physiology*, vol. 513, no. Pt 3, pp. 915–925, 1998.

9. M. Maskrey, D. Megirian, and J. H. Sherrey, "Alteration in breathing of the awake rat after laryngeal and diaphragmatic muscle paralysis," (in eng), *Respiration Physiology*, vol. 81, no. 2, pp. 203–12, Aug 1990.

10. D. R. Hillman and K. E. Finucane, "Respiratory pressure partitioning during quiet inspiration in unilateral and bilateral diaphragmatic weakness," *American Review of Respiratory Disease*, vol. 137, no. 6, pp. 1401–1405, 1988/06/01 1988.

11. S. Parthasarathy, A. Jubran, F. Laghi, and M. J. Tobin, "Sternomastoid, rib cage, and expiratory muscle activity during weaning failure," *Journal of Applied Physiology*, vol. 103, no. 1, pp. 140–147, 2007/07/01 2007.

12. M. Dres et al., "Usefulness of Parasternal Intercostal Muscle Ultrasound during Weaning from Mechanical Ventilation," *Anesthesiology*, vol. 132, no. 5, pp. 1114–1125, 2020.

13. N. Nakanishi, J. Oto, Y. Ueno, E. Nakataki, T. Itagaki, and M. Nishimura, "Change in diaphragm and intercostal muscle thickness in mechanically ventilated patients: a prospective observational ultrasonography study," (in eng), *Journal of Intensive Care*, vol. 7, p. 56, 2019.

14. Z. H. Shi et al., "Expiratory muscle dysfunction in critically ill patients: towards improved understanding," *Intensive Care Medicine*, vol. 45, no. 8, pp. 1061–1071, Aug 2019.

15. J. F. Brichant and A. De Troyer, "On the intercostal muscle compensation for diaphragmatic paralysis in the dog," (in eng), *Journal of Physiology*, vol. 500, no. Pt 1, pp. 245–253, 1997.

16. A. De Troyer and T. A. Wilson, "Mechanism of the increased rib cage expansion produced by the diaphragm with abdominal support," *Journal of Applied Physiology*, vol. 118, no. 8, pp. 989–995, 2015/04/15 2015.

17. J. Doorduin, L. H. Roesthuis, D. Jansen, J. G. van der Hoeven, H. W. H. van Hees, and L. M. A. Heunks, "Respiratory muscle effort during expiration in successful and failed weaning from mechanical ventilation," *Anesthesiology*, vol. 129, no. 3, pp. 490–501, 2018.

18. B. De Jonghe et al., "Respiratory weakness is associated with limb weakness and delayed weaning in critical illness," (in eng), *Critical Care Medicine*, vol. 35, no. 9, pp. 2007–15, Sep 2007.

19. W.-L. Su et al., "Involuntary cough strength and extubation outcomes for patients in an ICU," *Chest*, vol. 137, no. 4, pp. 777–782, 2010/04/01 2010.

20. P. Formenti, M. Umbrello, M. Dres, and D. Chiumello, "Ultrasonographic assessment of parasternal intercostal muscles during mechanical ventilation," *Annals of Intensive Care*, vol. 10, p. 120, 09/07 2020.

21. S. J. Cala, C. M. Kenyon, A. Lee, K. Watkin, P. T. Macklem, and D. F. Rochester, "Respiratory ultrasonography of human parasternal intercostal muscle in vivo," *Ultrasound in Medicine & Biology*, vol. 24, no. 3, pp. 313–326, 1998/03/01 1998.

22. R. Yoshida et al., "Measurement of intercostal muscle thickness with ultrasound imaging during maximal breathing," (in eng), *Journal of Physical Therapy Science*, vol. 31, no. 4, pp. 340–343, Apr 2019.

23. P. Wallbridge et al., "Parasternal intercostal muscle ultrasound in chronic obstructive pulmonary disease correlates with spirometric severity," *Scientific Reports*, vol. 8, no. 1, p. 15274, 2018/10/15 2018.

24. M. Umbrello et al., "Oesophageal pressure and respiratory muscle ultrasonographic measurements indicate inspiratory effort during pressure support ventilation," *British Journal of Anaesthesia*, vol. 125, no. 1, pp. e148–e157, 2020/07/01 2020.

25. N. Tahan, K. Khademi-Kalantari, M. A. Mohseni-Bandpei, S. Mikaili, A. A. Baghban, and S. Jaberzadeh, "Measurement of superficial and deep abdominal muscle thickness: an ultrasonography study," (in eng), *Journal of Physiological Anthropology*, vol. 35, no. 1, p. 17, Aug 23 2016.

26. A. De Troyer, M. Estenne, V. Ninane, D. Van Gansbeke, and M. Gorini, "Transversus abdominis muscle function in humans," (in eng), *Journal of Applied Physiology* (1985), vol. 68, no. 3, pp. 1010–6, Mar 1990.

27. G. Misuri et al., "In vivo ultrasound assessment of respiratory function of abdominal muscles in normal subjects," (in eng), *The European Respiratory Journal*, vol. 10, no. 12, pp. 2861–7, Dec 1997.

28. G. Rankin, M. Stokes, and D. J. Newham, "Abdominal muscle size and symmetry in normal subjects," (in eng), *Muscle Nerve*, vol. 34, no. 3, pp. 320–6, Sep 2006.

29. B. A. Springer, B. J. Mielcarek, T. K. Nesfield, and D. S. Teyhen, "Relationships among lateral abdominal muscles, gender, body mass index, and hand dominance," (in eng), *The Journal of Orthopaedic and Sports Physical Therapy*, vol. 36, no. 5, pp. 289–97, May 2006.

30. Z.-H. Shi et al., "Changes in respiratory muscle thickness during mechanical ventilation: focus on expiratory muscles," *Anesthesiology*, vol. 134, p. 748–759, 2021.

31. O. Rasouli, A. M. Arab, M. Amiri, and S. Jaberzadeh, "Ultrasound measurement of deep abdominal muscle activity in sitting positions with different stability levels in subjects with and without chronic low back pain," (in eng), *Manual Therapy*, vol. 16, no. 4, pp. 388–93, Aug 2011.

32. A. Reeve and A. Dilley, "Effects of posture on the thickness of transversus abdominis in pain-free subjects," *Manual Therapy*, vol. 14, no. 6, pp. 679–684, 2009/12/01 2009.

33. A. H. Jonkman et al., "Breath-synchronized electrical stimulation of the expiratory muscles in mechanically ventilated patients: a randomized controlled feasibility study and pooled analysis," *Critical Care*, vol. 24, no. 1, p. 628, 2020/10/30 2020.

34. K. M. Diab, A. Shalabi, J. A. Sevastik, and P. Güntner, "A method for morphometric study of the intercostal muscles by high-resolution ultrasound," *European Spine Journal*, vol. 7, no. 3, pp. 224–228, 1998/06/01 1998.

35. M. M. Ijland, J. Lemson, J. G. van der Hoeven, and L. M. A. Heunks, "The impact of critical illness on the expiratory muscles and the diaphragm assessed by ultrasound in mechanical ventilated children," *Ann Intensive Care*, vol. 10, no. 1, p. 115, 2020/08/27 2020.

36. L. Costa, C. Maher, J. Latimer, and R. Smeets, "Reproducibility of rehabilitative ultrasound imaging for the measurement of abdominal muscle activity: a systematic review," *Physical Therapy*, vol. 89, pp. 756–69, 06/01 2009.

37. C. Pirri et al., "Inter-rater reliability and variability of ultrasound measurements of abdominal muscles and fasciae thickness," *Clinical Anatomy*, vol. 32, no. 7, pp. 948–960, 2019/10/01 2019. https://doi.org/10.1002/ca.23435

38. M. Taghipour et al., "Reliability of Real-time Ultrasound Imaging for the Assessment of Trunk Stabilizer Muscles: A Systematic Review of the Literature," *Journal of Ultrasound in Medicine*, vol. 38, no. 1, pp. 15–26, 2019/01/01 2019. https://doi.org/10.1002/jum.14661

39. H. M. Wallbridge, Parry SM, Irving L, Steinfort D, "Reduction of COPD hyperinflation by endobronchial valves improves intercostal muscle morphology on ultrasound," *International Journal of Chronic Obstructive Pulmonary Disease.*, vol. 15, pp. 3251–3259, 2020.

40. J. M. McMeeken, I. D. Beith, D. J. Newham, P. Milligan, and D. J. Critchley, "The relationship between EMG and change in thickness of transversus abdominis," *Clinical Biomechanics*, vol. 19, no. 4, pp. 337–342, 2004/05/01 2004.

41. D. Bachasson et al., "Diaphragm shear modulus reflects transdiaphragmatic pressure during isovolumetric inspiratory efforts and ventilation against inspiratory loading," *Journal of Applied Physiology*, vol. 126, no. 3, pp. 699–707, 2019.

42. A. Flatres et al., "Real-time shear wave ultrasound elastography: a new tool for the evaluation of diaphragm and limb muscle stiffness in critically ill patients," (in eng), *Critical Care*, vol. 24, no. 1, pp. 34–34, 2020.

43. E. Soilemezi, S. Savvidou, P. Sotiriou, D. Smyrniotis, M. Tsagourias, and D. Matamis, "Tissue doppler imaging of the diaphragm in healthy subjects and critically Ill patients," *American Journal of Respiratory and Critical Care Medicine*, vol. 202, no. 7, pp. 1005–1012, 2020/10/01 2020.

44. E. Oppersma et al., "Functional assessment of the diaphragm by speckle tracking ultrasound during inspiratory loading," (in eng), *Journal of Applied Physiology*, vol. 123, no. 5, pp. 1063–1070, Nov 1 2017.

45. Q. Fossé et al., "Ultrasound shear wave elastography for assessing diaphragm function in mechanically ventilated patients: a breath-by-breath analysis," *Critical Care*, vol. 24, no. 1, p. 669, 2020/11/27 2020.

46. P. Linek, T. Wolny, A. Myśliwiec, and A. Klepek, "Shear wave elastography for assessing lateral abdominal muscles in thoracolumbar scoliosis: A preliminary study," *Bio-Medical Materials and Engineering*, vol. 31, pp. 131–142, 2020.

47. X. Wang et al., "Use of shear wave elastography to quantify abdominal wall muscular properties in patients with incisional Hernia," *Ultrasound in Medicine & Biology*, vol. 46, no. 7, pp. 1651–1657, 2020/07/01 2020.

48. K. Reimers, C. D. Reimers, S. Wagner, I. Paetzke, and D. E. Pongratz, "Skeletal muscle sonography: a correlative study of echogenicity and morphology," *Journal of Ultrasound in Medicine*, vol. 12, no. 2, pp. 73–77, 1993/02/01 1993. https://doi.org/10.7863/jum.1993.12.2.73

49. F. JimÉnez-Díaz et al., "Experimental muscle injury: Correlation between ultrasound and histological findings," *Muscle & Nerve*, vol. 45, no. 5, pp. 705–712, 2012/05/01 2012. https://doi.org/10.1002/mus.23243

50. A. Sarwal et al., "Interobserver reliability of quantitative muscle sonographic analysis in the critically Ill population," *Journal of Ultrasound in Medicine*, vol. 34, no. 7, pp. 1191–1200, 2015/07/01 2015. https://doi.org/10.7863/ultra.34.7.1191

51. B. Coiffard et al., "Diaphragm echodensity in mechanically ventilated patients: a description of technique and outcomes," *Critical Care*, vol. 25, no. 1, p. 64, 2021/02/16 2021.

12

Tissue Doppler Imaging of the Diaphragm

Eleni Soilemezi, Panagiota Sotiriou, Savvoula Savvidou, and Matthew Tsagourias

Introduction

Doppler ultrasound detects the frequency shift of ultrasound signals reflected by moving objects. Conventional Doppler techniques assess the velocity of blood flow by measuring high-frequency, low-amplitude signals from small, fast-moving blood cells. In contrast, myocardial tissue velocities are typically much lower than the conventional velocities of blood flow. Therefore, in Tissue Doppler Imaging (TDI) mode, the ultrasound system is modified with the use of both filter adjustment and gain amplification, to allow display of low-velocity signals generated by the myocardium and to filter out higher-velocity signals generated by blood flow (1). Since TDI measures the velocity of moving *tissue*, it can be applied to study motion characteristics of the primary respiratory muscle, the diaphragm.

TDI is performed in both pulsed-wave and colour modes. The main use of pulsed-wave TDI is to measure peak myocardial velocities. With colour TDI, a colour-coded representation of myocardial velocities is superimposed on grey-scale two-dimensional or M-mode images indicating the direction and velocity of myocardial tissue motion (1).

Ultrasound Technique

As with all ultrasound techniques, image quality remains an important determinant of the accuracy of measurements. TDI images are acquired with a phased array 2–4 MHz

DOI: 10.1201/9781003128694-16

probe, i.e., the cardiac probe of the ultrasound machine. The right hemidiaphragm is routinely examined, due to the limited acoustic window offered by the spleen on the left (videos 12.1a, 12.b).

- B-mode images of the hemidiaphragm are first obtained. The probe is placed in the subcostal position between the midclavicular and anterior axillary lines, and oriented medially, cranially, and dorsally to obtain a clear view of the middle or posterior third of the examined hemidiaphragm; the latter parts of the diaphragm are examined since they demonstrate greater motility compared to the anterior diaphragmatic part.
- When the TDI option is selected, a colour-coded map is superimposed on the B-mode image, demonstrating the direction and velocity amplitude of diaphragmatic muscle motion.
- The PW Doppler cursor must then be aligned parallel to the diaphragmatic tissue examined, since TDI will only assess muscle movement parallel to the probe beam. The smallest Doppler angle possible should be used; as with conventional Doppler, increasing the angle between ultrasound beam and examined segments will lead to underestimation of velocity.
- The gate of the sample volume is directed to assess the diaphragmatic region of interest and widened to incorporate the whole range of diaphragmatic motion, if possible. In some patients with large diaphragmatic displacement, some contamination of the TDI sample volume with liver tissue may be observed; however, it has been demonstrated that adjacent tissues move similarly with the diaphragm during quiet and deep breathing (2), so estimated velocities are still expected to be accurate.
- The velocity scale must be lowered to 5 cm/sec to match the lower velocity of the moving diaphragm compared with that of the beating heart.
- The Doppler gain may need adjustment to allow clear delineation of diaphragmatic tissue motion with the lowest background noise.
- Sweep speed also needs to decrease to 10 or 25 mm/sec.
- Depending on the type of ultrasound machine, additional modifications of the images may be possible; for instance, the smooth control option softens the appearance of the trace data, allowing the TDI waveform to appear as a single continuous line. However, despite improved visualization of the contour of the velocity signal when using this option, some signal loss will occur and the estimated peak values will be directly affected; therefore, when measurements on TDI images are performed, the use of such technique options must be stated (Figures 12.1a, 12.1b).

Video 12.1a Two-dimensional (B-mode) approach is first used to identify the middle-posterior third of the right hemidiaphragm; zoom function is then applied.

Video 12.1b Application of TDI in B-mode with colour flow mapping. The colour map indicates the contraction velocity in red (diaphragm is moving towards the probe) and the relaxation velocity in blue (diaphragm is moving away from the probe).

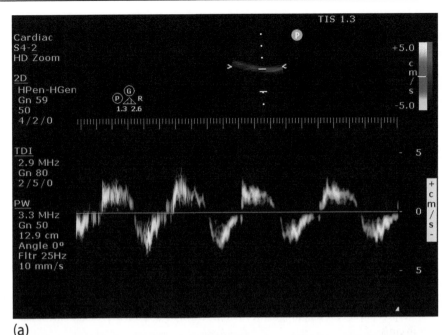

(a)

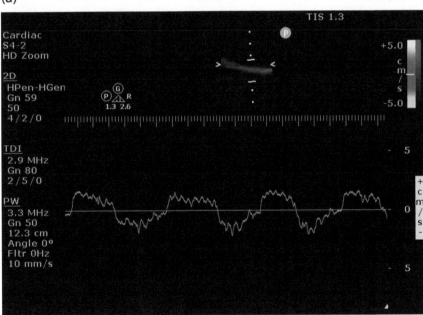

(b)

Figure 12.1 Diaphragmatic TDI in a healthy individual breathing quietly. Diaphragmatic TDI exhibits two waves, one during diaphragmatic contraction (above the baseline) and one during diaphragmatic relaxation (below the baseline). Depictions before (a) and after (b) applying the smooth control option of the sonographic machine are shown. Notice how the appearance and peak values change when this option is applied. Figure 12.1a was reprinted from (3), with permission of the American Thoracic Society. Copyright © 2021 American Thoracic Society. All rights reserved

All the modifications mentioned above can be saved as a preset ultrasound program, which, once selected, will incorporate all saved changes to avoid re-implementation of all the above before each examination.

The images acquired represent the depiction of the ***velocity*** (*y axis: diaphragmatic velocity, measured in cm/sec*) of the diaphragmatic motion over time (*x axis: time, measured in sec*), a feature of diaphragmatic muscle motion not widely studied so far.

Variables Identified

On each TDI waveform, we can identify and measure the following parameters (Figure 12.2):

- Peak contraction velocity (**PCV**), defined as the maximal diaphragmatic velocity during contraction, measured in cm/s;
- Velocity–time integral (**VTI**), defined as the area under the TDI curve during inspiration, measured in (cm/s)•s;
- Peak relaxation velocity (**PRV**), defined as the maximal diaphragmatic velocity during relaxation, measured in cm/s;
- TDI-derived maximal relaxation rate (**TDI-MRR**), defined as the slope of the initial steepest part of the diaphragmatic motion velocity curve during relaxation, measured in cm/s^2.

Use and Potential Applications

Ultrasound has been extensively used so far to assess diaphragmatic displacement, thickness, and thickening ratio. Diaphragmatic TDI, however, captures a different variable, the velocity, i.e., the speed of motion of the moving diaphragm. Limited literature exists to date to document the potential application of these recently described TDI-derived parameters in clinical practice.

- Recent literature suggests that healthy individuals and weaning success patients exhibit significantly lower peak contraction and relaxation velocities as well as lower relaxation rate compared to patients who fail to wean from the ventilator (Figures 12.3a, 12.3b, 12.3c). These high values of diaphragmatic velocities are most probably related to the shortening of inspiratory time and increased respiratory motor output, both well documented in patients who eventually fail weaning. Such observations raise the question of the potential use of TDI-derived parameters as weaning predictors. Such an option remains to be assessed; however, specifically for TDI-MRR the area under the receiver operator characteristic has already been studied and estimated as high as 0.80 (95% confidence interval, 0.71–0.89; $P < 0.001$) (3).
- In ICU patients in whom respiratory mechanics are studied with the use of trans-diaphragmatic pressure (Pdi) catheters, PCV is positively associated with the maximal value of Pdi during inspiration (Pdi peak), and also with the diaphragmatic pressure-time product (PTPdi) (3). This relationship is not unexpected, since in cardiac TDI, peak systolic velocities are related to left ventricular ejection fraction, therefore, they are used to quantify the systolic performance of the heart; similarly, Pdi peak and PTPdi represent indexes of diaphragmatic contractile performance.

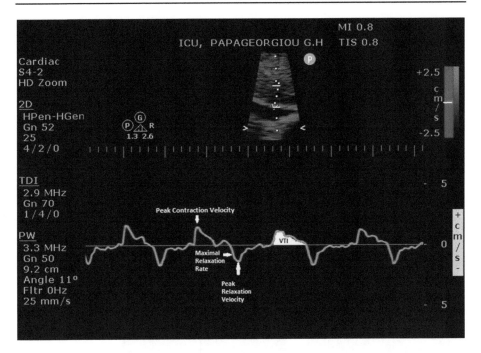

Figure 12.2 On each TDI waveform, the following parameters can be identified and measured: the maximal diaphragmatic velocity during contraction (peak contraction velocity); the maximal diaphragmatic velocity during relaxation (peak relaxation velocity); the area under the TDI curve during inspiration (velocity–time integral); and, finally, the slope of the initial steepest part of the TDI curve during relaxation (TDI-derived maximal relaxation rate). To more clearly demonstrate the points where measurements are performed, in this image we have used the smooth control option, which softens the appearance of the trace data, allowing the TDI waveform to appear as a single continuous line

- Diaphragmatic TDI allows direct, real-time assessment of the velocity and, also, the rate of change in the velocity, i.e., the acceleration or deceleration of the moving diaphragm, non-invasively, by the bedside. The maximal relaxation rate of the diaphragm during a spontaneous weaning trial has been of special interest to the intensivists, due to its prognostic value with regard to weaning (4). Until now there was no direct means to study the velocity of diaphragmatic motion, but it was assumed that changes in trans-diaphragmatic (Pdi) pressure reflect changes in diaphragmatic velocities. Accordingly, diaphragmatic maximal relaxation rate (i.e., a change in diaphragmatic motion *velocity*) was indirectly calculated as the slope of the descending part of the Pdi waveform) (i.e., from a change in *pressure*). Diaphragmatic TDI offers a direct and technically easier means of assessing the changes in diaphragmatic motion velocity; moreover, close agreement was found between the diaphragmatic relaxation rate acquired with the TDI technique and with the use of Pdi catheters, possibly allowing for implementation of the TDI technique in the assessment of the diaphragmatic relaxation rate during weaning. In addition to the relationship between TDI-MRR and Pdi-MRR, peak relaxation velocities also reflect diaphragmatic maximal relaxation rate, and may, therefore, be alternatively used for its assessment.
- In patients with neuromuscular disorders, sniff PCV was significantly reduced compared to controls and was correlated with FVC and sniff nasal pressure (5).

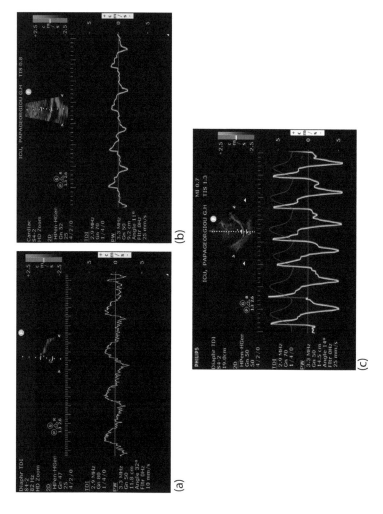

Figure 12.3 Figure 12.3a exhibits diaphragmatic TDI in a healthy subject breathing quietly. Note that the weaning success patient (Figure 12.3b) demonstrates a similar TDI pattern and similar TDI parameter values to those of the normal individual (technical note: the slight difference in appearance in the contour of the TDI waveform is due to the difference in the sweep speed used, 25 mm/sec in Figure 12.3a compared to 10 mm/sec in Figure 12.3b; a technical particularity of the specific ultrasound machine used). Conversely, a weaning failure patient (Figure 12.3c) shows a distinctively different pattern, mainly due to higher values of contraction and relaxation velocities and relaxation slope. Additionally Pdi waveform is depicted simultaneously to the diaphragmatic TDI one, revealing the positive correlation between PCV and peak Pdi. Figure 12.3c was adapted from (3), with permission of the American Thoracic Society. Copyright © 2021 American Thoracic Society. All rights reserved

Limitations of the Technique

As with all Doppler techniques, a disadvantage of TDI is the influence of the angle between the ultrasound beam and the investigated tissue motion, on estimation of tissue velocity. Moreover, TDI cannot distinguish between active muscle movement and passive displacement; therefore, recordings of diaphragmatic TDI in patients in assisted modes of ventilation must be interpreted with caution.

Future Directions

Diaphragmatic TDI is a new approach in the assessment of diaphragmatic tissue motion. Information is still needed regarding the determinants of diaphragmatic contraction and relaxation velocity, and larger studies are needed to delineate the Tdi pattern in patients who fail weaning due to different causes. However, the technique has an excellent reproducibility, tested both on adult (3) and neonate population (6), and provides a technically easy, real-time, by-the-bedside approach in assessing diaphragmatic motion velocity.

Key points

o TDI is a technique that allows recording of the velocity of moving tissue.
o When TDI is applied to the moving diaphragm, it allows real-time, direct assessment of the velocity of diaphragmatic motion during contraction and relaxation.
o Images of diaphragmatic TDI allow identification of the following variables: the maximal diaphragmatic velocity during contraction and during relaxation, the velocity–time integral, and finally, the TDI-derived diaphragmatic maximal relaxation rate.
o The future use of these recently described parameters in everyday clinical practice remains to be determined. A potential role in weaning could be possible since higher contraction and relaxation velocities are associated with worse weaning outcomes.

References

1. Ho CY, Solomon SD. A clinician's guide to Tissue Doppler Imaging. *Circulation* 2006; 113: 396–398.

2. Davies SC, Hill AL, Holmes RB, Halliwell M, Jackson PC. Ultrasound quantitation of respiratory organ motion in the upper abdomen. *Br J Radiol* 1994;67:1096–1102.

3. Soilemezi E, Savvidou S, Sotiriou P, Smyrniotis D, Tsagourias M, Matamis D. Tissue doppler imaging of the diaphragm in healthy subjects and critically ill patients. *Am J Respir Crit Care Med* 2020; 202:1005–1012.

4. Goldstone JC, Green M, Moxham J. Maximum relaxation rate of the diaphragm during weaning from mechanical ventilation. *Thorax* 1994; 49: 54–60.

5. Fayssoil A, Nguyen LS, Ogna A, et al. Diaphragm sniff ultrasound: Normal values, relationship with sniff nasal pressure and accuracy for predicting respiratory involvement in patients with neuromuscular disorders. *PLoSONE* 14(4):e0214288. https://doi.org/10.1371/journal.pone.0214288

6. Radicioni M, Rinaldi VE, Camerini PG, et al. Right diaphragmatic peak motion velocities on pulse wave tissue doppler imaging in neonates. Method, reproducibility and reference values. *J Ultrasound Med* 2019; 38: 2695–2701.

13

Ultrasound of the Diaphragm in Paediatric Patients

Massimo Zambon

In paediatric patients, the diaphragm is affected by a variety of diseases and conditions, such as congenital diseases, post-surgical phrenic nerve injuries, prolonged ventilation and atrophy, infections, tumours, trauma, and neuro-muscular disorders. Some of these entities are discussed in earlier chapters of the book and the ultrasound approach does not differ significantly from that utilized in adult patients. In this chapter some clinical entities typical of paediatric patients will be discussed, focusing on the role of ultrasound of the respiratory muscles in their management.

It is noteworthy that the diaphragm of the newborn is prone to dysfunction due to lower muscle mass, flattened shape, and decreased content of fatigue-resistant muscle fibres. This condition is worsened in premature infants [1].

- *Congenital diaphragmatic hernias (CDH).* CDH results from the inadequate formation of the diaphragm during embryogenesis and causes a cascade of events which can present in a newborn child varying clinically from mild to very severe to fatal. The incidence of CDH is 1 in 2,500 to 1 in 3,500 live births. The key to survival lies in prompt diagnosis and treatment. With the advent of newer surgical techniques for diaphragm repair, particularly the use of prosthetic patches, new complications and imaging appearances are seen. Furthermore, recurrence of hernia is a major problem and can be seen in 3–22% of cases. Patients with very large defects who require patch repair are at greatest risk of recurrence and other complications [2]. Prenatal sonography and MRI have allowed early and accurate identification of the defect and associated anomalies. In one multi-institutional study in Europe, the detection rate for CDH increased from 51% in uncomplicated cases to 72% when CDH was associated with other malformations [3]. Nevertheless, a CDH diagnosis can be challenging, as the clinical symptoms are often nonspecific, with radiographic findings potentially mimicking other chest conditions such as pneumonia, pleural effusion, and pneumothorax. An incorrect diagnosis may expose the patient to unnecessary or harmful interventions such as thoracostomy tube placement. The pattern of ultrasound for CDH diagnosis includes: (1) partial absence of the hyperechoic line representing the normal diaphragmatic profile, (2) partial absence of the pleural line in the affected hemithorax, (3) presence of multi-layered area with hyperechoic contents in motion (normal gut), and (4) possible presence of parenchymatous organs (i.e., liver or spleen) inside the thorax [4] (Figure 13.1).

DOI: 10.1201/9781003128694-17

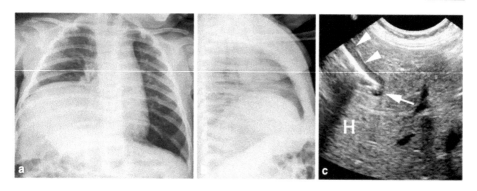

Figure 13.1 A 5-month-old boy, with late diagnosis of right Bochdalek hernia. The child presented with respiratory distress and fever. *a and b:* Anteroposterior and lateral chest radiographs demonstrate global elevation of the right diaphragm. *c:* Lateral long-view US (c) demonstrates the normal anterior hypoechogenic diaphragmatic muscle (arrowheads), partial absence of the hyperechoic line representing the normal diaphragmatic profile with the folding free edge of the diaphragm (arrow), and the herniated liver (H) (from [5] (with permission)

- *Paralysis or dysfunction due to phrenic nerve injury,* a well-described complication after congenital heart surgery, with an incidence ranging between 0.3% and 20% [6, 7]. Bedside ultrasonography has become the gold standard to diagnose diaphragm paralysis after paediatric cardiac surgery, with a sensitivity of 96.7% and a specificity of 96.15% [8].
- *Ventilator-induced DD.* As for adult patients, DD also occurs in association with critical illness neuromyopathy, or due to MV [9–11]. Diaphragm atrophy is present in children on mechanical ventilation for acute respiratory failure. In a recent study, Glau et al. demonstrated a 3.4% decrease in median diaphragm thickness per day of MV [12], a result similar to that found by Zambon et al. in adult patients [13]. The combination of exposure to neuromuscular blockade infusion with low overall spontaneous breathing fraction is associated with a greater degree of atrophy.
- *Bronchiolitis.* In recent studies, diaphragm ultrasound has been tested as a bedside tool for evaluation and outcome prediction of infants with bronchiolitis. It is straightforward that the assessment of respiratory muscles workload and the use of accessory muscle plays a major decisional role in the management of severe bronchiolitis [14]. Diaphragmatic excursion, inspiratory and expiratory slope were correlated with clinical severity scores [15, 16].

Ultrasonography has gained popularity as a modality that can be performed quickly and serially at the bedside. It allows not only to diagnose dysfunction or congenital diseases, but also to track the evolution of diaphragm function. In comparison to fluoroscopy, the diagnosis of DD with ultrasound is less time consuming, avoids radiation exposure in paediatric patients, and does not require transferring patients to a radiology suite.

Either for diaphragmatic thickness/thickening and excursion, the technique is essentially the same as that in adult patients, and as for adult patients, the right hemidiaphragm is usually better visualized than the left one [17].

In smaller patients, with an oblique transverse subxiphoid view obtained at the midline, it is often possible to visualize both diaphragm domes. Real-time comparison of movements of the hemidiaphragms can be performed to easily detect unilateral paralysis [18].

Measurement of maximal inspiratory excursion at TLC may not be viable in infants and young children, given their inability to cooperate.

Only a few small trials focused on healthy spontaneously breathing infants have tried to characterize diaphragm ultrasound parameters to determine reference values for excursion, thickness and thickening, and its evolution with age.

References

1. Dassios T, Vervenioti A, Dimitriou G. Respiratory muscle function in the newborn: a narrative review. *Pediatr Res.* 2021 Apr 19:1–9.

2. Chavhan BG, Babyn PS, Cohen RA, et al. Multimodality imaging of the pediatric diaphragm: anatomy and patho-logic conditions. *RadioGraphics.* 2010; 30:1797–1817.

3. Garne E, Haeusler M, Barisic I, et al. Congenital diaphragmatic hernia: evaluation of prenatal diagnosis in 20 European regions. *Ultrasound Obstet Gynecol.* 2002;19:329–333.

4. Corsini, I., Parri, N., Coviello, C., et al. Lung ultrasound findings in congenital diaphragmatic hernia. *Eur J Pediatr.* 2019;178, 491–495.

5. Gil-Juanmiquel L, Gratacós M, Castilla-Fernández Y, et al. Bedside ultrasound for the diagnosis of abnormal diaphragmatic motion in children after heart surgery. *Pediatr Crit Care Med.* 2017;18:159–164.

6. Sanchez de Toledo J, Munoz R, Landsittel D, et al. Diagnosis of abnormal diaphragm motion after cardiothoracic surgery: ultrasound performed by a cardiac intensivist vs. fluoroscopy. *Congenit Heart Dis.* 2010;5:565–572.

7. Parmar D, Panchal J, Parmar N, et al. Early diagnosis of diaphragm palsy after pediatric cardiac surgery and outcome after diaphragm plication: A single-center experience. *Ann Pediatr Cardiol.* 2021;14:178–186.

8. Banwell BL, Mildner RJ, Hassall AC, et al. Muscle weakness in critically ill children. *Neurology.* 2003;61(12):1779–1782.

9. Johnson RW, Ng KWP, Dietz AR, et al. Muscle atrophy in mechanically-ventilated critically ill children. *PLOS One.* 2018;13(12):0207720.

10. Valverde Montoro D, García Soler P, Hernández Yuste A, Camacho Alonso JM. Ultrasound assessment of ventilator-induced diaphragmatic dysfunction in mechanically ventilated pediatric patients. *Paediatr Respir Rev.* 2021 Feb 23:S1526–0542(21)00005–1.

11. Glau CL, Conlon TW, Himebauch AS, et al. Progressive diaphragm atrophy in pediatric acute respiratory failure. *Pediatr Crit Care Med.* 2018 May;19(5):406–411.

12. Zambon M, Beccaria P, Matsuno J, et al. Mechanical ventilation and diaphragmatic atrophy in critically Ill patients: an ultrasound study. *Crit Care Med.* 2016;44:1347–52.

13. Duarte-Dorado DM, Madero-Orostegui DS, Rodriguez-Martinez CE, et al. Validation of a scale to assess the severity of bronchiolitis in a population of hospitalized infants. *J Asthma.* 2013;50:1056–61.

14. Şık N, Çitlenbik H, Öztürk A, et al. Point of care diaphragm ultrasound in acute bronchiolitis: A measurable tool to predict the clinical, sonographic severity of the disease, and outcomes. *Pediatr Pulmonol.* 2021;56:1053–1059.

15. Buonsenso D, Supino MC, Giglioni E, et al. Point of care diaphragm ultrasound in infants with bronchiolitis: A prospective study. *Pediatr Pulmonol.* 2018;53:778–786.

16. Zambon M, Cabrini L, Zangrillo A. Diaphragmatic ultrasound in critically Ill patients. *Annual update in Intensive Care and Emergency Medicine.* 2013;2013:427–438.

17. Weber MD, Lim JKB, Glau C, Conlon T, James R, Lee JH. A narrative review of diaphragmatic ultrasound in pediatric critical care. *Pediatr Pulmonol.* 2021;56:2471–2483.

18. Karmazyn, B., Shold, A.J., Delaney, L.R., et al. Ultrasound evaluation of right diaphragmatic eventration and hernia. *Pediatr Radiol.* 2019;49:1010–1017.

Index

T - #0147 - 111024 - C168 - 234/156/8 - PB - 9780367652760 - Gloss Lamination